# Back ]
# *Permanent* Healing

## Understanding the
## Myths, Lies, & Confusion

# Steve Ozanich

Author of

**The Great Pain Deception:
Faulty Medical Advice Is Making Us Worse**

and

**Dr. John Sarno's
Top 10
Healing Discoveries**

Cover image and stock illustrations used under license from Shutterstock.com

ISBN: 978-0-9965866-0-3
1st Edition

Designed by Steve Ozanich
Cover layout and design: Taylor Krzeszowski
Photography: Michael Stephen Studios

Publisher:     Silver Cord Records, Inc.
               PO Box 8513
               Warren, OH 44484


SteveOzanich.com

Printed on acid-free paper

after breathing exercise

I am Strong          with hands
I +                  on
~~I am~~ healthy     tummy.

I am Safe ←

~~I am fine~~

There is nothing Seriously
Wrong with me. ←
                        Be Calmer
                        when
I am fine        Breath
                 5 Secs in
        For      5  "    "

## Dude and Peanut

*Let your minds thirst for Knowledge …*
*and your hearts drink from Truth*

You have to be calm first or
mind wont believe you...... before
you make a movement.

# Back Pain
# *Permanent* Healing

## Understanding the Myths, Lies, & Confusion

### Foreword by
### Paul Gwozdz, MD

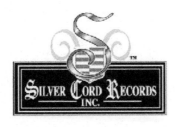

SILVER CORD RECORDS INC.

# Table of Contents

# Foreword

> *A truth's initial commotion is directly proportional to how deeply the lie was believed. It wasn't the world being round that agitated people, but that the world wasn't flat. When a well-packaged web of lies has been sold gradually to the masses over generations, the truth will seem utterly preposterous and its speaker a raving lunatic.*
>
> Donald James Wheal, (1931-2008)

American medicine has traditionally focused on diseases of the physical body and mind but has misunderstood the large role that emotions play in our chronic pain. The truth is in many cases, that emotions are the primary cause of our chronic physical pain. John E. Sarno, MD, discovered this in the mid-20th century, identified it as TMS, and proved it by successfully treating his patients at the Howard A. Rusk Institute of Rehabilitative Medicine at the New York University Medical Center. He educated patients that their back pain in most cases was due to psychological causes rather than physical/structural causes and he began having remarkable cures of chronic back pain!

According to Dr. Sarno, chronic pain can be caused by the unconscious mind, generating the pain as a distraction so that the patients would not have to think about the things that they did not want to think about. Testimonials regarding the positive effect of applying his theory are well documented in his four books and can be widely found on the web.

I credit Dr. Sarno for saving my life from one that would have destined me to sit in front of a TV while on disability and pain medications. But fortunately I didn't go that direction; instead I found his first little book *Mind over Back Pain* in the county library after being told by my orthopedic surgeon that my severe back pain was caused by my herniated discs and that there was nothing that could be done for me. After all, my MRI clearly showed that I had two herniated discs. I was still an engineering manager at the time and unhappy in my job. But once I was healed after seeing Dr. Sarno as a patient, I had the courage to leave my career and enter medical school at the age of 40. I am now a family physician and also a TMS doctor having trained under Dr. Sarno as an M.D. For the past 15 years, I have been seeing TMS patients from across the U.S. and overseas.

Many doctors, particularly specialists, look at the pain path at the tissue level and try to cure the body. The pharmaceutical industry looks at it from a molecular level and tries to develop drugs to diminish the pain. Physicians concentrate on MRI findings and often make faulty assumptions about the significance of them while ignoring the fact that many people with no pain have the exact same findings.

I have seen many patients use Dr. Sarno's techniques to heal, and by reading this book, *Back Pain, Permanent Healing,* many more sufferers will understand that their chronic pain may stem from unacceptable emotional conflicts rather than physical causes. Steven Ray Ozanich also discovered this through his personal experience.

After Steve wrote his highly regarded first book, *The Great Pain Deception*, he clearly established himself as a leading TMS expert. He then began having conversations with many people with chronic pain and listened to all of the excuses that these TMS patients used to prevent themselves from getting better. After all, many TMS sufferers think that they are outliers and cannot be cured.

Steve has taken the essence of these many conversations and put them down on paper. This book is truly a conversation with the patient who is not yet able to understand and accept their diagnosis of TMS. But it's also a book for any one with back pain who cannot find answers. It serves to clarify what Dr. Sarno teaches us and provides answers to naysayers regarding the myths that surround back pain. If you are cynical of both Dr. Sarno's approach, and of the back pain industry's approach to curing your pain, then this book is for you. It is also a good source if you just want to better understand TMS.

I want to emphasize how important having confidence in Dr. Sarno's teachings is to the healing process. Please note that I use the term "confidence" instead of "faith" since Dr. Sarno is not teaching religion. You may start out skeptical, but as you become more knowledgeable and work with the TMS concept, you will gain confidence that you too can be healed. Keep in mind that your brain is always ready to continue creating pain to help distract you from thinking about the things you don't want to think about. It is normal in the beginning of the healing process to default back to the medical pain model. It may take some time to understand and accumulate your own reservoir of evidence to totally accept Dr. Sarno's teachings.

Your TMS doctor or psychotherapist also needs to understand the difference between acute pain and chronic pain. It is imperative that they have an unwavering understanding and confidence in Dr. Sarno's model in order to increase your confidence that you can be cured. If your TMS diagnostician lacks confidence then you need to move on. Of course, you must always begin by seeing your physician to rule out a malignant process, but once that is done you can begin the path of healing.

The good news is that you can be healed of your TMS by reading this book because Steve so clearly rebuts many of the negative thoughts and arguments for why people cannot be cured. It is important that you use this confidence to your benefit so that you too can become pain-free.

Enjoy and good luck, and be ready to hear that the world is round when everyone knows that it is flat.

Paul Gwozdz, MD, New Jersey, USA

May, 29, 2016

# Acknowledgments

The first acknowledgment of thanks should always be given to Dr. Sarno, not only for his keen observations in healing, but also for his unwavering courage in publishing his findings. He is indeed a true pioneer in health and healing, the greatest pain doctor in the world. I, along with countless others, have been able to live a happier and more fulfilled life because of his deep desire to help. Not only has he helped masses of people heal around the world, but he also created new careers, saved relationships, expanded the sciences, enlightened the spirits, and forever corrected the false and archaic paradigm of pain. In the midst of his many great accomplishments he remains humble—a great professional, and greater man.

My sincerest gratitude to TMS physician Paul Gwozdz, MD, for taking the time from his hectic schedule to create a Foreword and in helping with the accuracy of the medical information contained in this book. He freely gave his time and advice from his own desire to help people, through advancing truth.

A special thanks to Joe Polish, founder of Genius Network, for his selfless help in spreading Dr. Sarno's beautiful healing message. You can have a great message but it doesn't mean anything if it falls in a forest where there's no one to hear it. Joe may be the busiest person in the world, but it hasn't slowed him from helping as many people as he can, from the generosity of his heart.

A huge thank you to Michael Galinsky at Rumur for standing tall on the front line of "the great cause," by being there to bounce ideas off of, and in helping to connect with others who want to help.

To Tom Fields, for his kindness in helping to keep the TMS message going with his generosity. And to Jane Barlow Christensen for her giving of her personal time and effort, and for her deep desire to help others understand this great message.

A heart-felt thank you to editor extraordinaire Karen V. Kibler, PhD, who learned me how to write gooder, and who soars far above and beyond the call of duty as a matter of her normal work ethic. And, to the best squeezer-book formatter around, Eric J. Fletcher, whom I haven't been able to stump when it comes to Word and its never-ending troublesome scenarios.

Thank you to those whose help has been priceless along the journey: Marc D. Sopher, MD, Andrea Leonard-Segal, MD, Peter Zafirides, MD, Jack Travis, MD, Margaret Chan, PhD, Kirsten Fliegler, PhD, Dan Hollings, Susan "She" Cyphers-Keener, Deborah von

Schuster-Reisdorf, Jackie "Jack" Chancey, Mayela "Bee" Gerhardt, Heather Zarella, Caroline "Cazz" Brown, Colly "Wally" James, Lara "LaLa" Held, Ana Stockwell, Ales Kezman, Natalie "Nats" Holdaway, Walter "Walt" Oleksy, Eric "Herbie" Watson, Greg Swenson, Lori "Lou" Losch, Allison Mains Beardsley, Tom Ross and the boys at Clear Choice Creative, Nelson Crain and Brad Kolasinski.

Thank you to Amy Duncan for her hard work in creating and maintaining a Facebook TMS group to help suffering people, and to Forest Smith for helping to gather important information; good people helping good people.

Thanks to Jungian Analyst Paul Benedetto, RP, for his kind help, and to the thousands of former pain sufferers who have reached out to contact me for help, and who shared their healing stories. I learn something from every one of them and they become part of my own story.

# The Rock

I am strong, my own reflection, I see a rock upon a hill
Change not says fear imprisons me, pretend ye to be still

I lay beneath the sun, pray lie within the storm
My shell can ne'er be broken, no noise when walked upon

I am, and who I think I am, cannot both agree
Held in doubt, turned inside out, imprisoned me by me

Colors flowered they surround me, all laughing with the sun
Tapped by the rain to dance the wind, they have all the fun

I've watched them laugh, and heard them play, but always will they wilt away
They grow and change, to light my world, but live to fade again today

Hands held within not felt nor failed, cold feet both never danced
Stone hardened I resist with strength, change not be dare not chanced

Chronic quiet seems to pacify, my supporting ground around
Silence screams to stop the voice, I cry I could have found

I reflect on inside out and back, a rock who should have tried
A pebble sitting endlessly, though whatsoever never died

I think I know, and thought I should, concealed within for all to see
My colors bloomed could light my world, if only I were free from me

**Shadow** *is the unknown, there are few things more frightening, and therefore resisted.*

Paul Benedetto, RP, Jungian Analyst

# Preface

**Back pain is not all in your head!!**
(There... I got it out of the way early on)

*We cannot change anything until we accept it. Condemnation does not liberate, it oppresses.*

CG Jung, MD[1]

I agonized through crippling back pain for nearly 30 years, until I discovered in the late 1990s that back pain almost never comes from defects in the spine's structure. Doctors led me to believe, at an early age, that my pain was coming from problems in my spine. That insidious notion caused me two-thirds of a life of suffering. Back pain rarely, if ever, comes from herniated discs or spinal narrowing, and it certainly doesn't come from spinal curvature, core weakness, slipped discs, or spinal misalignment. The latest scientific studies have disproved these archaic notions of back pain being caused by spinal "abnormalities." But, tragically, an entire mythology has already been built around this bogus terminology that has aided in unnecessarily crippling millions of people—and has made many more very wealthy.

I was repeatedly diagnosed with severe herniated discs at L4, L5, and S1, and told they were the cause of my pain. I was also diagnosed on many occasions with spinal stenosis (narrowing), and told that the narrowing was the cause of my pain. I was also diagnosed with spinal disc arthritis (osteoarthritis), and spinal disc spurring (osteophytes), as well as, disc degeneration (water loss). I was diagnosed as having one leg longer than the other, as the cause of my pain. My left leg was partially paralyzed at one point in 1990, with no tendon reflexes, and no sensation except for pins and needles. I lost over 50 lbs. from intense back pain in 1998, and at countless times was unable to walk, or stand up. For three decades I had been told that spinal defects were causing my back pain, but it was never true. These things are **superstitions; myths** that have been perpetuated by pain practitioners throughout various specialties, around the world. The ongoing back pain problems are exacerbated by the belief that the spine's flaws are causing back pain.

**Superstition:** *any blindly accepted belief or notion.*

**Myth:** *an idea that is believed by many people but is not true.*

Since I healed, I've helped thousands of people with so-called "bad spines" to free themselves from pain by restoring good health through education. In this book I'll explain:

- Why almost all back pain occurs;
- Why most sufferers would rather treat their back than get rid of their pain;
- Why there is so much confusion regarding back pain;
- Why "trying to heal" is the biggest mistake a back pain sufferer can make;
- How to eliminate back pain permanently without surgery, drugs, injections, or physical therapy—AND—why some people think these techniques worked, when the problem only shifted.

Back pain has now become the #1 cause of job disability in the world. Pain, in general, costs Americans annually approximately 600 billion dollars—both in medical costs and through lost productivity[2]. But the vast majority of these costs could be avoided, just as most of the suffering can be prevented. What sufferers don't know about pain is the very source of their pain. What many refuse to accept about their pain ... is the very cause of their ongoing torment.

In the 1970s, pioneering pain physician John E. Sarno, MD, revolutionized healing by uncovering the reason for almost all pain, including back pain, and through formulating a groundbreaking model for dealing with the cause of pain. He labeled the cause **TMS**, for **Tension Myoneural Syndrome**. This healing revelation has become such a powerful force within every aspect of health that TMS is now being referred to as **The Mindbody Syndrome**. It's one of the most brilliant discoveries in medical history, yet few people know about it, and fewer want to know about it. Nonetheless, healing takes place with this new knowledge virtually every single time, for those who want to heal, and are **ready**.

> *It should be emphasized that this book (Healing Back Pain) does not describe a "new approach" to the treatment of back pain. TMS is a new diagnosis and, therefore, must be treated in a manner appropriate to the diagnosis ... **clearly there is no logic to traditional physical treatment.** Instead experience has shown that the only successful and permanent way to treat the problem is by teaching patients to understand what they have.*
>
> John E. Sarno, MD[3]

# Introduction

The great back pain mystery was solved decades ago by New York University physiatrist John E. Sarno, MD. But there are pockets in areas around the world that haven't heard the news yet. Some haven't had the opportunity, and many who have heard reject the solution. And so daily, the pain industry, as well as the common back pain sufferer, continues on a gratuitous journey, seeking solutions for a problem that has long since been resolved.

If you go into any random back pain group or pain forum and offer up the advice on how to heal, you will summarily be scolded by group members, and occasionally kicked off the site by the site's administrator. Healing is rarely a welcomed message, except by a select few open-minded and "ready" individuals.* I have been a member of many such pain groups.

Sufferers don't normally gather at pain groups and forums to heal, they tend to congregate to seek out ways of coping with their pain, treating it, living with it, and sharing in the personal agony. Given the choice between treating their spine with a therapeutic technique or measure, and permanent healing, statistically most would choose to treat their spine. Healing is too often incomprehensible with current understanding. **Permanent healing** begins with the knowledge of *why the pain exists in the first place*, not from "how to" books, or magical words of advice from pain practitioners.

This is not a "what to do" to heal your spine book. This is a book on how to get rid of the cause of your pain, allowing the pain to fade away forever. There is no step-by-step program that can yield "real healing" for anyone, in the long run. There are many sources to go to that can provide temporary placebos. In fact, everything sufferers "are doing to heal" is the reason their pain won't stay away, but they aren't realizing this. I have witnessed healing occur in countless pain sufferers. They were all **ready** to give up "doing things to heal" and to find victory over suffering through deeper understanding.

---

*Pay close attention to the word "ready." It is the key word predicting when healing will take place. All who are ready to see and accept the reason for their pain will welcome this message of healing. Those who cannot absorb it will reject it. Through time and learning, all those sufferers who get to the point of "readiness," can heal ... permanently.

Permanent healing is not always the first conscious choice among most pain sufferers. They frequently prefer to first "try some form of" new pillow, mattress, physical therapy, injection, spinal manipulation, Prolotherapy, stretching, acupuncture, drug, or surgery—and most important—they are unaware that these varying treatments are causing their pain to stay in the long run. They are further unaware that every time they feel better after attempting such techniques, it is due to a placebo response. Their deep belief that the technique was actually helping made them temporarily feel better. But the pain returns because the cause was never addressed, the brain was simply fooled (diverted).

The possibility of lasting healing is rarely on the conscious radar for a complex set of reasons to be explained throughout this book. And what is not fully understood about TMS is often decried as dogma. The *understanding* of all the various myths, lies, and overall confusion surrounding the back pain pandemic *is the healing mechanism itself.* Dr. Sarno referred to the information, as to what's really going on as "... the penicillin to this disorder." It is indeed. The reasons for the mass confusion regarding what's working and what's not are now much clearer thanks to Dr. Sarno's identification of the cause/reason of back pain. But the confusion steadily marches on ....

I've had a dozen or so back pain sufferers approach me in local restaurants and at private gatherings to say, "Excuse me, but I was told you wrote a book on back pain?" I then explain to them about my recovery and how Dr. Sarno has helped at least hundreds of thousands of people to heal from back pain, and that my first book has helped at minimum 10,000 to heal (from the email responses only). Every one of those who have walked up to me has answered in a similar fashion, "That's great man, that is so cool, congratulations!" They then limp away—never even asking the names of the books, or how all those other people are healing. Healing is simply not considered by most who are in pain because:

1. They've been told by their healthcare practitioner that they have a flawed or defective spine. And—they've made the mistake of believing that professional.

2. Their back pain, unbeknownst to them, is protecting them from aspects of themselves, from something that they don't want to know, or admit to. So deep down they're not **ready** to relinquish their pain even though they don't want the pain. It is still serving its purpose for them.

**Permanent healing** from back pain requires courage, and a profound change in understanding, through a radically open mind. But, more important—people have to want to heal. That may sound odd, because sufferers don't want pain. But what they don't understand yet is that "they need" their pain. Within this need to protect their suffering through relentlessly defending a "flawed spine," they will often refute the process I'm going to describe. How do I know? I was exactly like them! I became irate when it was suggested that my pain wasn't coming from my spine's defects, and threw *Healing Back Pain** across my room. But I was wrong, too. Healing is not about getting rid of back pain; it's about taking away the reason for it. The pain has a very specific purpose of which the typical sufferer is unmindful.

Dr. Sarno proved, clinically, that almost everything that is currently accepted about back pain by both laymen and professionals is wrong. Lasting healing comes from a deeper understanding, and in rejecting the **myths** and **lies** born from **confusion** that grew into the #1 cause of disability on Earth.

 *Everything that I have concluded about this whole (back pain) business is based on what I have seen. There is not one arm chair conclusion in any of this ... (it comes from) hands-on work with thousands of patients.*

John E. Sarno, MD[4]

---

*Healing Back Pain* is the most revolutionary book ever written on back pain; the bible of TMS pain.

# 1

# The Seeds of Understanding

While he was an attending physician at the Howard A. Rusk Institute of Rehabilitation Medicine, at New York University Medical Center, Dr. Sarno noted that back surgery wasn't working; it was failing to bring effective relief to his patients. He also noted unsatisfactory results from physical therapy, as well as from steroidal injections, and all the other therapeutic techniques being commonly administered. He instinctively felt that there had to be something else going on with back pain. So he began to look more deeply into his patients' charts where he noticed that his back pain patients also had many other things going on with their health. In addition to back pain, many had bouts of shoulder and hip pain, knee pain, foot and hand pain, skin problems, anxiety, depression, migraines, ulcers, irritable bowel, heartburn, frequent urination, and allergies, etc. *Where there's smoke there's often fire.*

So he began to dig even more deeply into their lives through conversing with them; during his conversations with them, he observed that most of them were fairly conscientious people. Most were worriers—driven, slightly-to-highly anxious, polite, gentle, kind, people-pleasers, tough on themselves—more often responsible in their duties. The most significant trait he observed was that they were placing tremendous pressure on themselves **to be good people**. They leaned toward perfectionism which was dramatically elevating their **tension** levels. Their perfection was a byproduct of their personalities, formed in early childhood. Their spines were fine! They were holding deep anger, in the form of tension, in their backs, but they weren't aware of it. The abnormalities Dr. Sarno was seeing on their imagings were from a normal aging process, and were in no way causing their crippling pain.

He stated on ABC 20/20's, "Dr. Sarno's Cure," that the herniated discs and structural changes seen on the MRIs "couldn't in a million years produce the level of pain that people get with this syndrome," and yet—physicians were routinely blaming these natural changes for back pain. The physicians were actually making the sufferers' pain worse—by pointing to harmless alterations in their spines as the causes of their pain. We now know that these benign and natural changes do not produce pain. But a chief cause of the epidemic of chronic back pain is that each sufferer feels they are somehow the exception, that their pain is unique, and that they have a bad spine. This is almost never true, but the myth lives on because many doctors don't know about TMS; however, soon everyone will. *Darkness cannot stop light from spreading.*

The most important concept to understand in healing back pain is the **power of belief**. What you believe will determine how bad or how long you will suffer, or whether you will ever heal. We have been led to believe the wrong ideas about our spines; but thankfully, Dr. Sarno exposed those fallacies long ago.

> *... after a few years of making the conventional diagnosis and administering the conventional treatments, I came to the conclusion that there was something terribly wrong, because my results were as poor as everybody else's. I found this frustrating and decided I'd better take a closer look at this and really question the diagnosis.*
>
> John E. Sarno, MD[5]

During his search for better answers, the good doctor observed that these sufferers were experiencing deep conflict within themselves that was often masked by a markedly cool manner, a do-good persona, and strong repressive tendencies. They were usually nice people, but not always; often had experienced turbulent, tense, anxiety-ridden, or even traumatic childhoods, but not always. As adults, they were pushing themselves hard, juggling their current problems, trying to keep everyone around them happy. They wanted to be good people—good fathers, good mothers, good sons and daughters, good workers and students—pushing themselves in order to be liked, to succeed—pushing, pushing, pushing to do the right things. In the process, they had lost sight of their own needs, who they were, how they felt, and what they wanted—giving rise to a considerable unconscious struggle within—and anger! Within their struggle to maintain this **false-Self**, coordinated by a demanding persona, their surfacing emotions were attempting to be made known through their pain. Their back pain was the expression of an intense and unconscious emotional conflict that they weren't even aware existed.

Some of their childhoods were actually good ones, but they still harbored great tension for complex reasons. Much of their adult anxiety and resulting pain was the effect of a personality that formed from parents who were absent, expected too much of them, and from parents who they felt didn't provide enough emotional support—**as perceived by them**, as children.

## A Mind Divided

One of Dr. Sarno's many revolutionary discoveries is that this intense need to be good—to be a good person—is actually deeply enraging; infuriating to the point of creating deep unconscious turmoil *... and severe pain ....*

"Unconscious" means that sufferers don't know they're angry; angry to the point of rage. It's all unfelt (which is why most people deny being angry). Their back pain is the only sign that these powerful emotions even exist. If sufferers do sense any strong emotions within themselves, then they're not aware of their intense magnitude. Thus, any anger (rage) they do feel has nothing to do with their back pain because that anger is conscious, and so it is "felt." **It is the anger, rage, fear, sadness, and resentment that they cannot feel that is causing their back pain.** Their anger, fear, frustration, and sorrows are simply substituted for pain, by their brain, so that they won't feel these emotions. Their brain does this as **a favor to them**—to help them cope through their daily life, to keep them *perfectly unaware* of any conflict within themselves. Since they are not aware of any conflict, or of its intensity, they often deny the very notion of conflict. This denial is another favor performed by the brain for the sufferer. The deeper self does this for specific reasons, to be discussed throughout this book.

Most sufferers are under the impression that they're angry and frustrated "because of" their back pain—but it's quite the opposite. They have back pain because they're unconsciously angry—at trying to be something they're not, having to do things they don't want to do, and to bury events they don't want to remember. Dr. Sarno would later refer to this phenomenon of conflict as "the divided mind"; divided between the conscious attempts to be good and to please others and the unconscious aspects of the Self that are enraged at these attempts.

## The New Movement

Back pain is a mindbody effect.* Emotions from internal conflict are expressed in the form of pain because the sufferer doesn't realize, or won't consciously admit that any conflict exists. What is too overwhelming for her is diverted to her body by her ego, and so she never senses its presence, or its scope. **Back pain is almost always from an emotional process called TMS**—and the first step in healing is to accept that this is true. Denying back pain as an emotional process is itself a psychological **defense mechanism** against healing, which is why people have to want to heal in order to permanently heal.

---

*Refers to back pain that is not due to cancer, aneurisms, acute injuries, or infections, etc. But it's important to note that people also heal from pain with existing cracked vertebrae, infections, so-called "old injuries," and other odd abnormalities with this information. What is often thought to be the cause of pain is more often not the cause. Be responsible, get examined to rule out danger.

Temporary healing can easily be found through any modern placebo treatment (discussed later).

Dr. Sarno turned the world inside out with his keen observation that people unconsciously create their own pain in order to divert their awareness to their body, distracting them away from their thoughts, feelings, and emotions. His work is now spreading like a slow burning fire across the globe, lighting the darkness with truth along the way. In successfully unraveling the great pain mystery, he began to help people heal from every type of pain from back pain, to hand and foot pain, to knee and shoulder, and pelvic and hip pain. Sufferers came to him with the most difficult cases of pain and suffering, and he succeeded in helping them heal at an astoundingly high rate. But they had to first believe and accept that their spines were okay, despite what their imagings showed, and despite what their physicians had told them.

I am one voice of many testimonials to the truth of his work. However, TMS-healing didn't stop at pain—there was much more on the horizon, as people began to heal from many other health problems with this new knowledge. Dr. Sarno unraveled the great medical mystery regarding why people are so unhealthy.

*There are so many things little and big that are TMS that I wouldn't have time to write about all of them.*
John E. Sarno, MD, to patients

## The Desire to Heal

Here is where a great controversy was born. The source of back pain is not what the physicians are pointing to in the spine (but most people think it is) ... AND ... it's not imagined (which most people feel they're being told). Back pain is real, and it runs the gamut from nagging to crippling. However, it's a mindbody effect—originating in the mind, and permeating the body. More precisely, back pain emanates from the autonomic nervous system—not the spine. If you truly want to heal, I urge you to keep your mind open and learn about this process. It's the greatest gift you will ever give yourself. But you first have to stop defending your body's flaws as causing your pain. This is too high of a hurdle for many.

People are sometimes aghast when I tell them that in order to heal, they have to want to heal. They often proclaim, "I DO NOT WANT my pain!!" But I'm not talking about getting rid of pain. I'm talking about eliminating the reason for the pain. The reason for back pain is more dangerous to the sufferer than the physical pain, which is why their brain has substituted physical pain in place of emotional angst. And so, the reason for the pain needs to be recognized and healed, not the spine. Therefore, healing is not about getting rid of pain, it's about taking away the need for the physical diversion.

We're through the looking glass in understanding, as our awareness of what is truly occurring has been turned upside down through perceptive observation—followed by astronomical success. Dr. Sarno brought the world a new paradigm of understanding, and he should have won the Nobel Prize in Medicine for his discoveries. Nonetheless, he proved beyond any doubt that the physical pain originates from a mental process, and that it can be discontinued by a new mental process. Tragically, few sufferers believe this, which makes trying to help people a frustrating ordeal. Even so, those who accept the notion heal nicely. The proof of this is everywhere. Feel free to visit YouTube at "TMS Healing Wall of Victory – The Great Pain Deception" to see some beautiful outcomes.

The work of spreading the TMS message is highly rewarding when someone has the strength to open up to the concept, reject their old beliefs, ignore their doctor's crippling advice, and burns with a desire to heal. Healing comes through **awareness** and then **acceptance**, but first must come **courage**.

*With one lecture Sarno cured me of 20 years of back pain.*
John Stossel[6]

## Frustration in Helping People Heal

*Tell all the truth but tell it slant —*
*Success in Circuit lies*
*Too bright for our infirm Delight*
*The Truth's superb surprise*
*As Lightning to the Children eased*
*With explanation kind*
*The Truth must dazzle gradually*
*Or every man be blind —*

Emily Dickenson

Everyone comes to truth in their own time, except for those who refuse to see it, of course. But those who seek verity in healing will heal when they're **ready**. Dr. Sarno's revelations regarding TMS are self-evident. And yet, most sufferers reject the notion of back pain being from anything other than a bad back. However—it isn't only those who repudiate back pain as a mindbody effect who are struggling. Resistance also comes from those who want to believe in TMS, but are not quite **ready** to lower their protective shields. They'll often say to me,

"I was a bit scared after talking to you, wondering what I would do if I actually healed." Their healing time is nearing because they're beginning to see who they are and why they have pain. When their hearts are **ready** they will heal; and when the patterns they fall into become more intelligible to them. Sometimes it's effortless to see who will heal nicely and who is going to struggle, based on their early actions, and words. The number one sign that someone is **not ready** to heal is when they trash the TMS message. Other common signs they're **not quite ready** are evidenced by the following actions:

- They throw *Healing Back Pain* across the room.
- They want free help only.
- They search for discrepancies in the TMS materials to find something to dispute, to exclude themselves as potential candidates for healing, often proclaiming, "Not everything is TMS!"
- They impugn the motives of those who are helping people heal.
- They never act on the TMS information in front of them.
- They ask questions to which they already have the answers.
- They jump from one TMS expert to another.
- They hear but don't listen.

Often when I'm explaining TMS to a person debilitated by pain, we end up talking past one another. Their eyes are often intense with expression, and their heads nodding quickly, waiting for me to stop talking about my dumb TMS topic so that they can tell me about their bad back. They're not aware that I'm explaining to them how they can heal. They've been told for so long, by so many, that they have a bad spine that they become part of their own disability in a dreadful self-fulfilling prophecy. It's not their fault, though; the bombardment of false memes has for so long imprisoned them inside a paradigm with no windows to see out of. These poor folks would no doubt listen if they felt there was hope.

There are also *unconscious defenses* against healing which will be discussed a few pages later, and an infinite number of ways to delay the inevitable outcome of healing. But nothing is as problematic as rejecting truth. Sometimes sufferers will ask me if their spouse or mate can sit in on a consultation. But when they do, their partners never agree on how the sufferer sees themselves. In fact, I can't remember one single instance, on personal topics, where they have agreed. The sufferer says something, and the partner shakes their head as if to say, "No way!" A couple of them have even retorted to the suffering spouse, "Who are you??" This usually involves how they think they react to life, or how they see themselves, or other people. How they view themselves is part of the larger picture of not being true to Self. Notwithstanding any inaccurate self-perceptions, these people can heal, and they do heal when they are **ready**. In the meantime, the truth behind their pain needs to be portioned out slowly and delicately or they tend to turn off quickly.

People are sensitive beings who do not like their feelings hurt, or their beliefs and values challenged. The truth, as it is, must sometimes be told slanted, to avoid even greater resistance. How a message is delivered is as important as the message itself.

I see healing as a type of Truth Template that needs to be placed over sufferers' lives, in order to heal those wounds they have rejected from awareness. To heal, the template needs to align properly with their memories, thoughts, and actions. But they also have to want to align their lives with who they truly are. Once they do, they have healed.

## Proof of Truth

When the wounded ones understand and accept "why" they have back pain, they **begin** to heal. The process I'm describing in detail has already worked in hundreds of thousands, and more likely in millions of people. I regularly receive calls and emails from ecstatic people, from every walk of life, who have healed. Most had spent years dealing with back pain experts, agonizing through various sorts of unnecessary medical procedures. They're all free now. But I didn't heal them—I'm not a healer. They freed themselves with insight, and renewed belief. I provided the blueprints, from Dr. Sarno who was the architect, but they had to construct their own temple of healing.

And healing they are! People are healing virtually every day, but they dare not tell their loved ones and friends for fear of reprisal. Once a sufferer heals, they're so excited to help other sufferers that they can hardly contain themselves. They want to share the peace and joy of what they have experienced, and of how they healed. But they're routinely met with ridicule, sarcasm, and disbelief. Former sufferers are sometimes hesitant to openly talk about being pain-free because they get chastised for the way in which they did it. You would think that someone suffering in great pain would be interested in learning how someone else healed from the same type of pain? Not so much.

Healing comes from within; it's the only way, but is despised by some as nonconformity against science. The end result is a denial and separation from truth, which guarantees continued suffering. Science doesn't determine Truth, it only reveals it. Truth already is.

## Ichthys  ⟨⟩✕

I've been contacted by pain scientists and practitioners from three prestigious pain centers to say that they were amazed as they watched chronic pain patients healing "right before their eyes" with my first book, which is based on Dr. Sarno's work. They had been unable to do anything for the sufferers. The tragedy is that I can't even mention the scientist's names because they're all in fear of adversely affecting their careers. One pain clinician stood behind a plant in her office and whispered to thank me on her cell phone for fear of coworkers hearing how she healed, which was by stopping the very remedies her pain clinic was advocating.

TMS physician Marc Sopher, MD, relayed a story to me that he was sitting in a waiting room with three ladies who were openly talking about their back pain. Naturally, the ladies weren't aware that Dr. Sopher (who trained with Dr. Sarno) had already helped many people heal from the back pain they were experiencing, and from their conversations it was apparent that they all had TMS. In a related email he said to me, "I didn't say a word to them, Steve, because you know how that would have ended."

Helping people heal is a touchy subject because many will rigorously defend the notion of a flawed spine and body, and also is why so many are disgusted with the current medical system. Money defines the current paradigm of healing, and most systems are set up to treat and manage pain, not to eliminate it. What does pain management even mean? Why would anyone want to manage their pain? Managing pain means controlling it, or coping with it. With Dr. Sarno's work, we can eliminate pain permanently by taking away its purpose.

On the flip side—the joy of watching people heal is indescribable. It immensely outweighs the backlash of trying to help. But that's okay; not only did I once feel that treating my spine was the correct way to heal, most of the former sufferers have felt the same way, at first. I'm not pointing a finger at anyone in particular, or pointing with any particular finger. I'm simply relaying what I've experienced from doing this full time for the past 16 years, to anyone who wants to heal. It's grindingly tough to deliver such a controversial message, and, you have to have a thick skin to handle the repercussion of criticism in explaining the great successes—but the dry, methodical work to spread truth continues.

## The Essence of What's Really Going On

Dr. Sarno came to the irreproachable conclusion that virtually all of his back pain patients were holding powerful emotions in their body, in the final form of tension—from unconscious anger generated from fear, as well as other strong emotions such as frustration, resentment, and deep sadness. And they were completely unaware of the continuing influence of these emotions on their health, oftentimes of their very existence.

The sufferer's brain reduces the blood supply to the spinal muscles and nerves, **on purpose**, to distract him from his surfacing and unwanted emotions. Thus he no longer feels the full brunt of his emotions as his physical pain substitutes for their full sensation. With agonizing pain now dominating his every waking second, he is forced to obsess on his body, and away from its emotional cause. As long as his brain can fool him into believing his pain is from a failing spine, his conflict and needs remain hidden in his body. He never knows they exist. He is only aware of his back pain now, which is his brain's frantic intent—to make him think that his body is damaged. It's a foolproof strategy by his brain, but the tables are quickly turning through awareness.

Back pain is a great deception: a diversionary strategy of survival, by design. The whole ruse works as long as sufferers keep going to their doctors and the doctor tells them that they have some type of physical problem. Doctors, and various pain-specialists in numerous healthcare fields, are directly involved in not only initiating back pain with absurd warnings, but in prolonging suffering. The spinal problems are NOT problems—unless the sufferer **believes** them to be a problem. Believing they have a spinal issue keeps the sufferer in agony by not only increasing tension through increased worry, and allowing for the ongoing avoidance of the emotions—but the body will also adapt to match the misplaced belief. This means that the brain will continue to withdraw blood to the spinal nerves if the person believes the spine to be flawed. *The biology adapts to match the deeper conviction of the individual.*

One of the many keys to healing is to stop obsessing on, and treating, the spine: the spine is okay! But, the sufferer has to believe that it's okay or his brain will continue to accommodate his inaccurate belief.

*As long as he (the sufferer) is in any way preoccupied with what his body is doing (by thinking about his back, or trying to heal it), the pain will continue.*

John E. Sarno, MD[6]

This is the reason chronic back pain sufferers can't find a permanent solution. They're looking to resolve the problem through fixing a spine that doesn't need to be fixed. I can remember dozens of former sufferers who have relayed to me the same story: "When my doctor pointed to the herniated discs on my MRI, my back pain dramatically increased!" Some have said that their doctor used the mouse cursor to circle a herniation on their MRI, or that the physician stated the all-too-common and tragic phrase, "There it is! There's your problem right there, you're gonna need these discs trimmed, they're pinching your nerves!" Based on what we know today, the disc trimming is medical malpractice. But doctors keep doing it ... because no one can stop them from stating a wrong opinion.

# 2

# It's a Bloodflow Problem, Not a Spine Problem

When the brain reduces bloodflow ever so slightly, oxygen doesn't get delivered, and a devastating pain occurs. It's the same general concept as a cramp, heart angina, or a migraine, and it can be just as agonizing and debilitating. And regarding TMS, sufferers are subconsciously doing it to themselves so that they can cope through times that are stressful, go to places they don't really want to be, and deal with people who are emotionally demanding of them. Some will proclaim, "But I love my job ... I want to go there!!" But these people aren't aware of the divided mind and its many implications. They're trapped in the world of, "What I see is all that there is." But there's more ... much more.

*In each of us there is another whom we do not know.*

CG Jung, MD[7]

One of the many obstacles to believing in TMS is that the pain feels so structural that sufferers instinctively think that it's a physical problem. **The reduced oxygen to the nerves makes it feel very mechanical.** But that's what the brain wants the sufferer to think, to make them worry about their body. The obstacle is then raised much higher when their physician tells them that they indeed have a structural body problem. Everyone is fooled this way, at first, but the tide has quickly turned on this outdated thinking.

Pain is the accommodating brain's way of helping the person persevere through periods when self-imposed pressures become too much, and anxiety too high. The brain produces pain to prevent them from feeling the emotions. The physical symptom is a stabilizing force that allows the sufferer to slow life down when it's moving too fast by grounding the internal conflict to the corporeal body. In this elegant process, the sufferer looks calm on the outside, appearing in control to outside observers. Regrettably, in the conflict and confusion, the innocent spine gets blamed. The proof that the spine is not to blame is that the sufferers all heal once they cast aside all archaic notions of back pain.

## Specious Stew: Combinations of Meaningless Numbers

Adding even more bewilderment to the tragic misunderstanding of events is that sometimes the brain reduces bloodflow at the exact site of a herniated disc, or arthritis, or at the same level of disc narrowing, causing greater confusion in what is a **spurious correlation**—which means a *false association*.

Back pain is routinely attributed to common herniations, crooked spines, spine weakness, osteoarthritis, and spinal narrowing. But we know in lengthy retrospect that these irregularities almost never cause pain. The "notion" that they do cause pain is the very thing causing the pain—increasing the pain's intensity, and forcing it into chronicity due to the awesome power of the physician's archetypal influence, coupled with the sufferer's deep desire to believe in the physician.

> Her brain wants her to think that her pain is from her spine's flaws ... her doctor then tells her that her pain is from her spine's flaws, and she wants to believe in her doctor. Voila! A recipe for disaster stew.

## Painful Errors

> *In my experience these things (disc narrowing, herniated discs, disc bulging, stenosis, etc.) do not cause back pain.*
> John E. Sarno, MD, personal correspondence,
> and everywhere

In 2012, Forbes Magazine published two articles on Dr. Sarno, labeling him "America's Best Doctor." He is indeed the greatest pain doctor America has ever seen, but as the aphorism states, *no good deed ever goes unpunished.* A large percentage of people despise his message of "how to heal." And from my own experience in helping people permanently rid their pain, it's at this point in the explanation that it must be re-stated: **Your pain is NOT in your head**. Your pain is not imagined; it's very real, and as the good doctor described, "... it could produce more severe pain than anything else I knew of in clinical medicine[8]." However, TMS back pain is harmless. Many of the defects seen on the x-rays and MRIs are actually preventing back pain, not causing it.

A spinal stenosis study released in 2014 by Pekka Kuittinen, et al. in BMC Musculoskeletal Disorders showed that people with moderate stenosis had more trouble walking than sufferers with more severe stenosis. And there was no correlation between the stenosis on the imagings and back and leg pain. In the discussion section of the study it states, "The main finding of our study was that there is no linear correlation in the radiological degree of severity of LSS (Lumbar Spinal-Canal Stenosis) and clinical findings. In contrast, according to the visual evaluations of the central canal LSS, leg pain measured by VAS (Visually Assessed Severity) was higher in the moderate stenosis group than in the severe stenosis group."

Regarding back pain, the MRI findings mean almost nothing. But even more revealing in this Kuittinen study is that the worse the MRIs looked, stenosis-wise, the less pain the people were in, and the longer they could walk without pain. This led the study's designers to conclude that the worse the spines looked, the better the person was. The malformations being blamed for back pain by most doctors may often be preventing pain, not causing it. In the conclusion of the study it states, "Our findings indicate that advanced degenerative hypertrophy may potentially be a protective mechanism that causes relief of patient symptoms[9]."

Dr. Sarno discovered this decades ago. The imaging findings mean little, but such studies as these are ignored; sufferers don't want to hear it. But the reason that they don't want to hear that their spines are okay is yet another of Dr. Sarno's great discoveries.

In attributing natural spinal changes as the cause of pain, there has been great injury done to multitudes of sufferers, and an industry based on false assumptions has flourished. The pain industry has failed to solve any problems, but has profited greatly from the confusion—that it alone continues to create. It's somehow presumed that herniations and other spinal abnormalities cause back pain. But there's not one single ounce of proof that they do. In fact, the opposite is true. All current evidence points toward the fact that these spinal imperfections do not cause pain. Anyone interested can look at the dozens of studies, including the Jensen study from 1994, "Magnetic Resonance Imaging of the Lumbar Spine in People Without Back Pain[10]," which concluded that back pain and disc herniations are "coincidental findings."

**Coincidence:** *a striking occurrence by* **mere chance** *of two or more events at one time.*

Waleed Brinjikji, MD, and colleagues, conducted meta-analysis of 33 articles (See Appendix E) on over 3,100 people with lumbar disc abnormalities, but who had no pain. The scientists noted that the findings of disc degeneration, disc signal loss, disc height loss, disc protrusion, and facet arthropathy are "part of normal aging and not pathologic processes requiring intervention." They concluded by stating, "These findings suggest that many imaging-based degenerative features may be part of normal aging and unassociated with low back pain, especially when incidentally seen"[11]. So here we have three dozen studies disclosing that spinal disc "abnormalities" do not cause back pain, and not one single study in the medical literature showing that herniated discs (or other spinal malformations) do cause back pain. And yet, people in general have chosen to believe the unproven side, the very same people who demand scientific proof of TMS.

Herniated discs do not cause back pain. The brain will "sometimes use" the herniations as the source destination of the rage in order to more deeply convince the sufferer that she has a spinal problem. More often, the pain at a site of disc herniation is a coincidence. There are many similar study conclusions on various other areas of the human body. However, all the proof in the world cannot convince a person who needs a diversion, and who wants to believe there's something wrong with her body.

> *There's such a strong cultural mindset that the only legitimate way of treating disease is by giving drugs, and when you talk about using a mindbody treatment as a way of dealing with pain, it just is inconsistent with that prevailing medical model. I've never met Dr. Sarno. I've seen miraculous results of people I've sent to him, some results from people who have just read his books.*
>
> Andrew Weil, MD[12]

In short, Dr. Sarno's unparalleled success **proved** that the vast majority of back pain is due to an unconscious tension process. He blew the lid off the old fallacies with his successes in healing back pain. Even though the truth began unfolding in the 1970s, the work of spreading it is really just beginning because of the manner in which we now communicate with one another. The exact number of people who have healed is unknown because many prefer not to deal with the recrimination when explaining how they healed. So they remain silent.

This book is but one source for anyone interested in ending their suffering, one of a host of many wellsprings of TMS stories from former victims who have healed from severe back pain.

Over the past 16 years that I've been involved in spreading this beautiful healing message, I've seen violent repudiations, eye-rolling disgust, mocking laughter, incredulous denials, and blank-stared disbeliefs. I've been yelled at, spat at, and had things thrown toward me—all from trying to help. The naysayers look down on the people who have healed from TMS as though they were dumb, naïve, even confused. But it's perfectly the opposite. The people who refuse to see this truth are the ones who don't get it, and they view people who have healed from crippling pain as some type of cultists. There is indeed a cultist mentality involved but it's on the "structural side" of the argument.

The "spinal problem believers" are forever lost in suffering. The physician with higher credentials firmly convinces them they have a defective body. At that point, that's it—their healing has been negated. But what the physician doesn't know is harming them. Even worse, few physicians care to know.

> *99.999 percent of the medical profession does not accept this (TMS) diagnosis.*
>
> John E. Sarno, MD[5]

## The Dilemma

Henceforth—the competitive line has been drawn between:

---

The **structuralists**: Who believe back problems come from a failing spine.

*... AND ...*

The **mindbody** group: Who know the spine is simply expressing unfelt emotions.

---

However, the most subtle damage to the healing message comes from those who say they believe in TMS, who claim to be champions of mindbody healing ostensibly, but continue to treat people through therapeutic means. The structuralists can easily be ignored; they remain increasingly marginalized by overwhelming evidence. But those who claim to be mindbody practitioners but also continue to recommend surgery, and injections, and physical therapy, etc., do the most harm because they betray the full light of truth, thereby confusing and perpetuating suffering. Back pain is the #1 pain epidemic because of confusion. If people knew the fuller truth, through a unified message, chronic back pain would be a distant memory.

> *I'm convinced that Dr. Sarno is right and that all chronic back pain should be considered TMS until proved otherwise.*
>
> Andrew Weil, MD[13]

I receive healing stories from people almost every week, and yet others say it's not possible; and the naysayers are the ones not healing. There's no **logical** reason to reject something that can alleviate pain, but there's a "psycho"-logical reason. This is important! The word "psycho" is part of the contentiousness because people have sensitive egos. Some would rather live in pain than accept the healing solution. **Ego** in its most dominant state protects current self-image at the cost of suffering. Many immediately see mindbody back pain as a weakness, a threat to *persona*. But that's never true. Back pain as a coping mechanism is utilized by the strongest people. They accept the pain rather than harm anyone, or offend anyone, and to be able to fulfill their duties.

## Knowledge Is Power

*(After talking to Dr. Sarno) ... all of a sudden the (back) pain was gone, it was the closest thing I've ever had in my life to a religious experience, and I wept.*

Larry David, creator of "Seinfeld"
and "Curb Your Enthusiasm"

When Dr. Sarno began to explain this unconscious tension concept to his patients, some of them began to heal. The **knowledge** of what was occurring within them had actually begun to dissolve their pain, despite the wild things seen on their MRIs, and despite their doctors telling them about the urgent need to operate. This was **proof** that the pain was not coming from the harmless defects in their spine. So, why would someone not want to believe in TMS, not want to try it? Good question! It doesn't appear to make sense to reject something that can take suffering away. Or does it? In rejecting TMS, and holding firmly to the notion of a damaged spine, the sufferer is able to continue to disown his shadow. The "dis"-owning of his shadow allows him to deny his emotional pain, and unhappiness, and to remain as a helpless victim of what he prefers to believe is bad luck, or poor genetics. In accepting the lie, the truth is destroyed and suffering is the byproduct.

The psychological defense mechanisms of **denial**, **displacement**, **resistance**, **reaction-formation**, and **TMS** are helpful tools in protecting us from being overwhelmed, and in shielding us from aspects of our lives that we don't want to see. They are also quite complex to understand. My own observation, and experience, has awakened me to see that some people still need their pain; otherwise, they would never reject advice that would certainly help them. Sadly, they often have to become much worse before they'll open up to what's really going on.

I, too, kept rejecting this healing information, repeatedly, until I had fallen far enough to hit bottom. It was from the bottom that I was forced to finally look up. I lost over 50 pounds, couldn't walk, stand, or sit without searing pain. When I finally got bad enough, I decided to take a look at Dr. Sarno's work, anew. I'm now grateful that my pain got worse. It forced me to look deeper, and to open my mind to what was happening. The fall is sometimes necessary in order to have something to rise above; the deeper the fall the higher one can rise. Suffering itself is a powerful catalyst for change.

It's easily understandable why a spine surgeon would not want to hear that spinal surgery is almost always useless. They study hard through difficult years, enduring intense medical training, and they make a good living performing surgery. They're also well respected, which means they are not going to easily admit that they've been performing unnecessary operations. If you mix in the ingredient that they truly think they're doing good for their patients, you get a group of people who are not that interested in a non-surgical solution to pain. The only spine surgeons and orthopedic surgeons who believe in TMS (that I'm aware of) are the ones who were once in great pain themselves, and healed with Dr. Sarno's work. If they hadn't been in pain, and desperate, they would never have considered pain to be a powerful mindbody effect. Some of those surgeons are now writing their own books on TMS.

The same is true for chiropractors; few are going to want to know that spinal manipulation is unnecessary without an epic fight for survival, in a continuing struggle for respect. As for the rest of the pain industry, why would anyone readily risk their current income and stature when they believe in their heart that what they're doing is beneficial? From their perspective what they're doing is meaningful, which is why change, through deeper understanding, occurs slowly, if at all. This book is an attempt to shed light on a confusing topic in the hope that some will see deeper, follow the large numbers before them, and heal.

There will always be folks with a vested interest in their own interests, of course. But when they also wield the societal power of their professional credentials, they become part of the problem. Para-doxically, in the case of TMS, society has handed authority of its healthcare over to the very people who are harming its collective health. The problems stem from believing that everything they advise is true.

Our bodies are more often reacting to the pressures and demands we place on ourselves to be good people. The act of medicalizing the body into good health is simply playing into the hands of the deceitful ego's strategy, since we can never doctor away our relationship problems.

Healing requires that the advice from the various pain professionals be ignored, whether it's the newest life-changing study, current in-vogue sticking, stabbing, poking procedure, or latest fad technique. In too many ways, these procedures thrive on keeping people needlessly in fear. This is not to say that the health professionals are always wrong. They're not always wrong. They can be lifesavers under the correct circumstances. But a key driving force in the confusing mess is that each back pain sufferer feels as though they are the exception to the rule, and that they indeed have a real spinal problem, when they don't. Their spinal discs are no worse than the tens of thousands who have healed before them. Their sacral joints, osteoarthritis, spinal curvature, leg length, hip height, disc degeneration, or spinal narrowing is nowhere near as bad as many of the sufferers who have already healed from TMS. The intensity of their pain convinces them that they are unique. The avenue to healing is to become aware of what's going on— understand and accept—and then to seek balance. Included within the many defense mechanisms is the personal **psychological resistance** to accepting TMS as the cause of back pain.

There are many factors contributing to why you haven't heard of something called TMS, and to why you may be in pain right now. Every pain practitioner feels as though they have the answer. So we end up with a myriad of measures to alleviate back pain, but only one of which is working on a steady basis. And that one is by far the most controversial. The only thing we know for certain is that none of the mainstream approaches are effectively working; thus, the continuation of rising pain epidemics.

# 3

# The Case for TMS

*I was just in agony all the time ... I finished the book (Healing Back Pain), and I was running on the beach ... and I had been struggling to walk.*

Jonathan Ames, author/TV producer[12]

When you suddenly realize "why" your pain exists, it all becomes clearer as to why TMS is so controversial. And you can't permanently heal without also understanding the controversy. The controversy itself is the very reason there's been no good solution. But now Dr. Sarno has uncovered the reason for pain, as well as the reason for the controversy. **The pain has a protective purpose.** People don't WANT their pain—they NEED it. Their life is in such a current state of hidden imbalance that they need a diversion in which to hide their anger, bury their fear, neglect their worry, and ease their frustrations. If they are trying to be good people, and worry about using other diversionary obsessions such as drugs, alcohol, and gambling, etc., they will often turn their need for a diversionary obsession toward their body.

**Need:** *a necessity arising from the circumstances of a situation.*

My goal here is to lay out the evidence in order to allow sufferers to make a cogent decision for themselves. Whether you believe what I'm explaining here or not, it still works, virtually every single time. I've also heard every imaginable argument against it; and yet, people still continue to heal. What harm can it do for anyone to try it? I'll preface all responses by reminding everyone that I didn't believe it either. I understand their skepticism. But happily I was wrong. And I'm certainly going to be attacked for trying to help people because the nature of darkness is its absence of light. To protect themselves from the true cause of their pain, many will reject the solutions before them. One method of rejecting healing is in attacking the messenger. But helping people from agony is worth the backlash after seeing so many free of pain and happy again.

Who doesn't heal with TMS-healing?—those who don't believe it, and also the much rarer few with serious emotional abandonment trauma. I hear quite often, "Dr. Sarno makes a good case, but here's where he's wrong ...." They then go on to state something that's profoundly untrue in order to defend a defenseless position. TMS healing is an esoteric process that only a select few are **ready** to see, and accept. *The emperor has no clothes.* You either see it, or you don't.

## The Options

Currently, the world of healing back pain can be divided into three main approaches, or three leading opinions: **MIA, MDA,** and **DSA.**

1. **Medical Industry Approach, MIA**: Those who believe back pain is the effect of a physical, structural spinal problem that stems from defects in the spine, and its surrounding anatomy, and believe it can only be healed by scientifically engineering the spine "back" into good health, using external measures. This includes surgery, physical therapy, injections, manipulations, strengthening, stretching, etc. This group treats back pain, usually in perpetuity. Support for this opinion is rapidly fading.

2. **Multidisciplinary Approach, MDA:** Those who believe in the application of a myriad of modern medical techniques; e.g., *the kitchen sink approach.* This opinion believes in trying combinations of everything, and anything. Supporters of this approach feel that what works for one person may not work for another. Its slogan is "one size does not fit all." So, try 'em all—and see which one works for you! It thrives on multiple placebo responses and substantial confusion. This opinion is currently popular.

3. **Dr. Sarno's Approach, DSA:** Those who know that back pain is caused by powerful and hidden emotions. This group heals, without surgery, drugs, injections, or physical therapy. It's the fastest growing opinion in the world, and the most contentious. However, history teaches us that any truth that first comes to light is always met with great resistance—passing through the stages of ridicule, aggressive opposition, and eventually into final acceptance as being true, and axiomatic. This opinion is rapidly gaining popularity with the advent of the Internet, social media, and from the ever-increasing anecdotal stories of people who have healed.

So which group is right? I recently had a medical doctor say to me, regarding doctor Sarno's work, "Just because these people are healing doesn't mean TMS works!" I was so shocked by how nonsensical that statement was that I couldn't figure out how to respond to it. I'm not sure I've ever heard anything more illogical. Permanent healing is the ONLY thing that matters! If it's working almost every time, then it probably works.

However the optimal means in which to properly answer the question of "which method is correct" is to observe the outcomes in healing. Do we want to stick with a method, or methods, that are constantly failing, but that are considered "the proper way?" Or, do we want to utilize methods that are actually working?

> *Dr. Sarno has cured thousands of sufferers of chronic pain that the medical community has misdiagnosed and been unable to relieve ... It is a puzzlement to me how a doctor who produces dramatic beneficial results for his patients at little or no cost could be considered controversial whereas practitioners of costly, ineffectual so-called mainstream medicine are somehow regarded as more legitimate.*
>
> Edward Siedle, Forbes[14]

## The Evidence: (is) MIA

In 1994, within the US Department of Health and Human Services and in what is now called The Agency for Healthcare Research and Quality, an article was published on the ineffectiveness of back surgeries entitled, "Understanding Acute Low Back Pain Problems." The survey concluded that 1 in 100 back operations were successful, and that surgery often created more problems. That's a 99 percent failure rate. This coincides with Dr. Sarno's earlier observations, and is generally true. One surgery usually leads to multiple failed surgeries, because people normally refuse to give up on fixing their body. The surgery simply feeds the need to fixate on the body, which is what the brain wants the sufferer to do. But that's not the epitome of failure. Things can always be worse.

In my research, I was introduced to two people who had 10 back surgeries, each. That is the epitome of failure. The two had no interest whatsoever in healing with anything other than some type of procedure. They were locked onto their obsession strongly because the abandonment trauma behind their pain was simply too great to recognize. It needed to be rigorously and persistently diverted to their backs for their psychological safety. Their brains were doing an excellent job in helping them—keeping them unaware of the magnitude and roots of their personal rage by providing them with a diversionary target to attack.

> *... to the last I grapple with thee; from hell's heart I stab at thee; for hate's sake I spit my last breath at thee.*
>
> Herman Melville, *Moby Dick*

Their backs had become their white whale, their life revenge, a lifelong obsession to be focused on, and vilified. What they don't realize is that their preoccupation on correcting their spine is precisely what their brain wants ... AND ... precisely why they've been wholly unsuccessful with their surgeries. Their fear, anxiety, childhood memories, life traumas, rejections, low esteem, frustration, panic, and rage are projected onto their own backs. The obsessive fixation on repairing their spine **is helping them** to remain unaware. It does so by preventing them from experiencing the intensity of their emotions—providing them a specious, focal target (their spine).

 They feel pain instead of: fear, sadness, resentment, anger, and panic.

When offered a way out of suffering, their anger and frustration can shift toward the TMS message. It all makes superb sense once you understand The Mindbody Syndrome—especially after you've healed. You'll also begin to see the genius in Dr. Sarno's work. He was not only brilliant in his observations, but he was also courageous to challenge the standards. For what is genius without courage?

*Genius is talent set on fire by courage.*
Henry Van Dyke, author, educator, (1852-1933)

## The Brain's Favor

Obsession is a means by which our brain avoids certain aspects of life that are too emotionally painful. We obsessively focus on one thing in order to avoid something that's more distressing. **Obsession is a coping strategy; it eases fear.**

 Chronic back pain is OCDing: both are used to alleviate anxiety.

Our brain presents us with "gifts for coping" by protecting us from overwhelming fear and rage, and other powerful emotions, by utilizing various methods to divert the anxiety generated from emotions. One such method is OCDing. People perform repetitive acts to alleviate anxiety; the repetition of the act prevents and protects them from feeling overwhelmed.

Regarding back pain, the repetitious act is the thinking of the pain hundreds of times per day. Instead of cleaning her kitchen floor repeatedly, or checking and rechecking her locks and doors, her mind's eye shifts back and forth to her back, in order to ease her worry. Her "act of obsessing, thinking, and talking about her pain" helps her to better handle her anxiety. Once diverted, she never feels all of her anxiety; and so, she vociferously proclaims that anxiety doesn't exist in her, and that she's not angry.* If her pain was to be removed, by actually healing, she would have to suddenly face those thoughts and emotions that her pain is vigorously trying to help her avoid. So, of course, her first reaction to the notion of a mindbody cause of pain must be heavily refuted with vigor. The ruse of a bad back must remain in place for her psychological safety. She dare not even lift the lid of Pandora's Box for fear of exposing all its far-reaching consequences. She does this by stating how dumb the idea of TMS is, how it's not supported by science, how Freud is dead, that TMS is "too New-Agey," and that her back pain "is real." She throws every excuse at the very thing that can take her suffering away from her ... because she **needs her physical pain**. Her brain is protecting her.

 The deeper aspect of the psyche knows exactly why it has created the pain. There's no way it's going to easily give up the diversion without a fight. It "fights" by ignoring and discrediting any solution that may permanently remove the pain: Pandora's Protective Lid.

The brain diverts unwanted thoughts and emotions through any means available. One of the means of diversion is to **create bodily symptoms** such as back pain, allergies, sinus infections, skin problems, dizziness, fatigue, heartburn, etc. It's quite ingenious of the survival self, but it's necessary because people have to live together. They can't act on their darker thoughts and threatening emotions for fear of rejection, and further isolation.

## Stress Versus Tension

We can't always have what we want, when we want it, and so we repress to get along, and to be good people. Whenever we don't get what we wanted we experience **stress**. Stress is the difference between what "we wanted" versus "what we just got." Therefore, stress is a perception in the psyche which then creates **tension** in the body. Therefore stress is psychological, in the mind, and tension is physical, in the body. The two go hand in hand to create physical sensations. When we don't get what we think we want, we then indirectly get physical tension.

The pain is the expression of how we want to feel, but don't, what we want to say and do, but can't. The pain itself is the diversion of the

---

*Anxiety is anger that is not expressed.

expression of want. Hence, most of our suffering comes from the **desire of want**, which grows from a **perception**.

We all need something(s) to focus our problems away from whenever life threatens to overwhelm us. It's a survival response:

> **Surviving**: by either denying (blocking awareness through repressing) or by diverting (shifting awareness). Some people use drugs, gambling, OCD, workaholism, alcohol, eating, texting, gaming, extreme fitness, and an infinite variety of other obsessive fixations to alleviate their anxieties. Those who focus on their spines use back pain. Back pain is an unconscious, psychological, covert mechanism for coping, and it's highly effective because back pain has been sanctioned by collective societies as being acceptable to possess.

When a repressive limit is breached, the brain finds ways to express the overload physically because physical symptoms are okay to have in most current societies. Contrarily, emotional problems are often seen as taboo: shameful. We can call into work and say, "My back went out, I won't be in tomorrow." That's okay; people understand, and accept that problem. However, few people would consider calling into work to say, "I'm afraid, I won't be in tomorrow." The difference is in the shame, the most painful of all emotions because it isolates us.

Pain is legal, and moral, but it's also an addiction. The mind's eye peeks at the pain throughout the day to help the sufferer cope, by avoiding.

## Choosing Your Poison

We all need help in our lives with welcome distractions when our ego feels threatened by the sensation of being overrun.* Much of the time, we consciously choose our diversions such as yoga, alcohol, smoking, drugs, gambling, jogging, sex, music, breathing techniques, etc. These are coping strategies that are **conscious choices**. However, there are unconscious means to help us cope, as well. These are

---

*I've often been asked what I mean by "feeling overwhelmed, or overrun." One example would be depression. In many instances people get severe back pain when they're depressed. The pain prevents them from knowing they're depressed by diverting their awareness to the physical sensation; binding it to their awareness through obsession. So the sufferer never feels depressed, the brain has successfully done its job by keeping them unaware of the depression, or its intensity.

referred to as **defense mechanisms,** which are utilized when **superego becomes too demanding**. The list is lengthy, but the more common unconscious defense mechanisms include:

- **Repression:** Casting unwanted thoughts and emotions into the body; ego prevents unacceptable thoughts from entering awareness.

- **Projection:** Pointing out others' flaws so that your ego can deny that you, too, have those same flaws. In this way ego avoids guilt and shame. Calling someone a liar helps you to feel as though you have never lied.

- **Reaction Formation:** Adhering to the opposite impulse. Fawning over someone you hate.

- **Intellectualization:** Thinking, rather than feeling, when feeling becomes too painful. Given a frightening diagnosis a person may turn to gathering details of the medical treatments to assuage the feeling of fear.

> *If a man is perfect in his thinking he is surely never perfect in his feeling, because you cannot do the two things at the same time; they hinder each other.*
>
> CG Jung, MD[15]

- **Conversion:** Expressing psychic conflict as a physical symptom. Extreme stress transforming to numbness, seizures, inability to speak, etc.

- **Denial:** Blocking the truth by taking a stance against it. Denying that smoking is bad for health.

- **Displacement:** Redirecting the rage. Yelling at your kids because you hate your job.

- **Sublimation:** Satisfying an impulse in a socially acceptable way. Running a marathon instead of cheating on your spouse.

- **Regression:** Going backward in psychological time, relapsing into the innocence of infantilism to feel safe, secure, loved. Reverting to childlike behavior such as playing with toys, running to parents after a marital fight, becoming clingy to someone like a child, etc.

The list of defense mechanisms is long, but we can also unconsciously "catch" our means of escape according to what is currently acceptable, defined by what others around us are doing, suffering from, emitting. By mimicking them we "connect," which is our most basic need—to feel connected. *If we mimic or become them, they can no longer reject us. We hide within them, reflecting us in them, and them in us.*

Others give us "unconscious permission" to use certain diversions. By them having it, it's not as shameful. Ailments such as common stomach problems and dizziness, anxiety, sleeplessness, and repetitive behaviors are all **TMS equivalents**, in that they can provide a desperately needed distraction. The methods that our brains choose to help us cope are not always by our choice, but are observed by our senses. Back pain is the number one acceptable reason people miss work, in the entire world. What goes around comes around, but is not always our consciously chosen coping means.

**Diversionary:** *tending to draw attention away from the principal concern.*

Currently, many kids are diverting their personal anxieties through technology addictions, such as texting and gaming. In order to avoid rejection, many simply put their earbuds in to shut out the world, and along with it all of its problems. They bury their faces in their cellphones and iPads: they utilize "things" that will never criticize or reject them (unless the battery dies). What they don't realize is that they're not solving their problems; they're only pretending they don't exist.

## The High Water Mark

> *They go in and take out the herniated material, and they think they're doing something wonderful because they're attributing the (back) pain to that. Anything that can be seen as abnormal on x-rays, MRIs and so on, will be seized upon by the medical profession because they have no concept whatsoever of a psychosomatic process.*
>
> John E. Sarno, MD[12]

In the spring of 2014, the Annals of Rheumatic Diseases published findings that back pain had become the #1 cause of job disability in the world[16]. There have also been periods during which back pain was increasing 14 percent faster than the general population. How could any of the current standard methods of treating back pain be correct when the problem worsens? The reason the medical industry approach isn't working is that they're focusing on the wrong sources—AND—few people are paying attention to the fact that it isn't working. Apathy has added to the greater problem as sufferers normally just go along with whatever their healthcare providers tell them they need. But as the aphorism repeatedly states: *Insanity is doing the same thing over and over and expecting different results.*

> *It's funny, all you have to do is say something nobody understands and they'll do practically anything you want them to.*
>
> JD Salinger, *The Catcher In The Rye*

## Wagging the Dog

On the brightest side, Dr. Sarno had a healing rate well above the 90 percent range. His patients were screened, which means that they were checked for real problems like cancer, infections, tumors, or aneurisms. And they were verbally questioned on whether they were open to the notion of TMS. Healing is **totally dependent on belief**. Contrarily, if you believe your body is broken, then it is; and it will usually stay that way until the realization of why it hurts.

But even more impressive is that the good doctor saw the worst cases of back pain, the ones that had been failed by the medical industry and multidisciplinary approaches. He saw most of his patients **after** they had **tried everything else** because they simply refused to admit that their pain wasn't structurally based. Eventually, after repeated failed procedures, when their pain became too great, and they were desperate for relief, they began to open up to the possibility of an emotional cause. They were **ready**. I did the same thing. I hit rock bottom before I decided to heal. It's reminiscent of "The Story of The Howling Dog." A passerby sees a dog sitting and howling:

> **Passerby**: *Why is your dog howling?*
> **Owner**: *He's howling because he's sitting on a nail.*
> **Passerby**: *Why doesn't he just move then?*
> **Owner**: *Oh ... because it's not THAT bad.*

From 1998 to now, in 2016, I have seen this scenario too many times. Sufferers will seek scientific measures that repeatedly fail. Crossing their fingers and rolling their dice—aspiring that the next technique will suddenly end their suffering. Deep within, they hope that the "medical act" will bypass the problem, like the teenager on the cell phone. If the pain isn't debilitating, but simply nagging, they accept it, to live with forever. They walk with limps, favor one shoulder over the other, fear to pick anything up—and use all sorts of medical aids to help them mobilize. It's sad, and there's plenty of blame to go around for the misunderstanding. However, the good news is that people are healing once they discover TMS. And it doesn't matter how long they've had their back pain, or how many surgeries they've had. I received an email from a man who discovered TMS, and healed his back pain after 44 years (breaking my record of 30 years). Who says you can't teach an old howling dog new tricks?

## Quick Fix Versus True Healing

Several frustrated folks suffering severe back pain had been in contact with me regarding TMS healing, and then suddenly caved in and tried surgery. After surgery, when their pain became worse, deep guilt settled in. They emailed me saying they were distraught and disappointed in themselves for doubting TMS. Their wish had been that they may be the extreme case in which surgery would work. They were desperate, wanting to heal immediately, perhaps hoping to peek inside Pandora's Box without fully opening the lid. I felt sorry for them because I know how pain can skew rational thinking. But nothing good comes easily, and you can't cut fear away with a scalpel.

The reasons for confusion and resistance to healing are certainly complex, but my goal is to help people free themselves. Most of the problem with accepting the true cause of back pain is that the sufferers' doctors are supplying them with erroneous information about their pain, such as, "You need this and that ... OR ... you have this or that." There was a great article in the Wall Street Journal, by H. Gilbert Welch, MD, entitled, "Why the Best Doctors Often Do Nothing[17]." Dr. Welch made the point that the fear of losing patients by not "doing something" initiates a knee-jerk reaction by many physicians into prescribing unnecessary remedies such as testing, medication, or referrals to specialists. Many physicians feel inclined to come up with an answer for the sufferer, and so they make things up. This occurs quite a bit with fibromyalgia, and other man-made disorders like carpal tunnel syndrome, complex regional pain syndrome, pudendal neuralgia, iliotibial band syndrome, piriformis syndrome, reflex sympathetic dystrophy, and a host of other arcane phraseologies and diagnoses.

> *Doing something is a quick way to make patients **feel heard**, even if it is a poor substitute for actually having the time to listen. But we also feel pushed to act because many patients have been taught to believe that the good doctors can reliably fix problems by trying medications, ordering tests, and referring to specialists ... That leads to knee-jerk medicine ... Doctors can fix some problems, others are better fixed by the patient. Some problems will resolve on their own, others are better left alone (particularly those "problems" that don't bother you). The good doctor is not the one that always recommends doing something. It's too easy for the physician— and it's too easy for you to get somewhere you don't want to be ... Recognize that the doctor who advises **no action** may be the one who really cares for you.*

H. Gilbert Welch, MD[17]

A couple dozen or so folks contact me every year who have been diagnosed by their physicians as having "fibromyalgia disease"—telling the frightened patients that "there's not much you can do about it … there's no cure, you need to learn to manage it." Once they receive this devastating news they rapidly decline to the point that they have trouble walking and getting out of bed. Their physicians make them dramatically worse, sending them into severe pain and depression with a nonsensical diagnosis, and an ominous prognosis. When the fibro-sufferers contact me, I explain to them that they're physically all right, and that fibromyalgia is a doctor-perpetuated problem like carpal tunnel; the effect of an unconscious emotional process. If they accept that they're okay physically, they begin to heal immediately, reversing the damaging diagnosis, because their fear is substantially reduced. They then have to reflect on issues such as their childhood, and begin the process of understanding why they need a physical diversion at this time.

Doctors too often create fear where none is justifiable, through poor advice.

Some sufferers take longer to heal than others due to complex factors, but the healing begins as soon as they understand that they were given an inaccurate diagnosis. Former First Lady Eleanor Roosevelt said, "No one can make you feel inferior without your consent." The same holds true for accepting frightening diagnoses. If people believe their physician, they get much worse. If they reject their physician's advice, they tend to get much better. But the controversy over fibromyalgia is as heated as the one over back pain, even though the fibro sufferers also heal if they accept that their body is okay. However, it's best to leave the fibromyalgia debate for another time. In 1861, Abraham Lincoln urged the release of two Confederate envoys by saying "One war at a time," when British forces threatened to attack from the Canadian border, furious over the seizing of their envoys from the British steamship Trent. But the fibro war is coming soon, as well.

I'm not blaming doctors for purposefully doing wrong. This is not a blame game that one side can win over the other. Everyone is losing, except the profiteers. This is about helping people through awareness. Most doctors simply don't know about TMS, and are truly attempting to help their patients. But it can't be overstated—the main reason that back pain has become a worldwide pandemic is that sufferers feel that everything their doctor tells them is true. In the case of almost all pain, the doctors are wrong. They're inadvertently harming people, every day, by handing out faulty diagnoses. This is the **nocebo effect** (Latin, definition *"I will harm"*).

## Heal the Pain: Stop Treating the Body

The world is infected with multiple epidemics of confusion. Out of curiosity, I looked at Amazon's top 100 books in the category of "back pain." Dr. Sarno's *Healing Back Pain* was ranked #1 in its category, at that time. It's the best and most successful back pain book ever written. However, #2 in the ranking (at that time) was a book by a pain specialist whose book was stating the exact opposite message of Dr. Sarno's book. Hence, the book ranked #1 in the category of healing back pain, and the book ranked #2 in healing back pain were extolling the complete opposite messages; and both books were selling great!

The primary message of the pain specialist's book is that healing from back pain requires realigning the spine into its "primal posture." Dr. Sarno's experience and vast clinical success proved that you never have to do that to heal. I've also never seen anyone who needed postural realignment to heal, and neither have the TMS physicians. It's no wonder people are so confused. The truth gets mixed and clouded and twisted and muddled with pieces of truth, obfuscating the full light of truth. I can state with absolute certainty that back pain does not come from the misalignment of the spine, nor does it come from a weak or crooked spine. These spinal conditions are incidental findings to pain; the claims are myths, adding to the confusion.

**Incidental:** happening as a result of something else.

> *Eradication of microbial disease is a will-o'-the-wisp; pursuing it leads into a morass of hazy biological concepts, and half-truths.*

Rene Dubos, PhD[18]

A will-o'-the-wisp is something imaginary and elusive that misleads hope. A will-o'-the-wisp simply means, "It ain't gonna happen." The same notion Rene Dubos put forth is proving true for spinal problems; pursuing them from a medical/structural standpoint has only led to a bunch of confusing concepts, and half-truths. This is of course always countered by supporters of these methods with, "Everyone is different. What works for one person may not work for another." Statements like these are statements of defeatism. People, structurally, are very similar. They differ only by the magnitude of their emotions and personal experiences, and by how they have chosen to hide their true self. Anyone feeling better from procedures to correct spinal crookedness has experienced a **placebo** reaction. Their deep belief temporarily pleased them.

I experienced many placebo reactions, on many occasions, pre-Sarno. But every day health practitioners are telling people they need to lose weight, and to get stronger, and that they have one leg shorter than the other, and that they need a firmer mattress, and that they have a vitamin deficiency, etc. ... and there will always be people who go out and lose weight and stretch and strengthen and realign their core, and take a supplement, and temporarily heal—BUT—not "because of" these things, rather because:

- They deeply **believed** these rituals worked. Some have claimed that antibiotics helped alleviate their back pain. It probably did ... but only because they believed it would.

- These rituals built great **confidence in them**, they felt better about themselves afterward, and their backs feel better, *incidentally*.

- These rituals temporarily **diverted** their focus from their obsession on their back. Physical therapy itself diverts awareness from the pain, and onto the goal of healing, fooling the deeper self into thinking it has been "cured."

- They deeply believed in the **person** who told them to perform these rituals. That person connected on a professional and personal level, with great confidence in the ritual, and so the ritual has a more powerful healing influence.

- They finally had **hope** within the ritual—a direction.
  - ✓ They then relate their easing of symptoms to the placebo ritual (a spurious correlation), and they live in constant fear of hurting themselves again, as the confusion and the pain and the epidemics continue—all because there's nothing wrong with their spine, or their posture.

## Confusion Drives Current Reality

People can find false correlations everywhere if they try hard enough. Actor Jim Carrey did a movie on this concept called "23." The film is based on the obsession that all incidents are connected to the number 23: some form of, or permutation of 23. This, too, is a method of defense and diversion and coping: *the searching*. We can find causal relationships in anything, if we search for them. But it's often just **apophenia**: *a psychological condition of the seeing of patterns in meaningless or random information and data, and then assigning meaning to the unrelated events.* But as we look deeper we can see that it's just dumb and dumber to force correlations where they don't exist, and to try to quantify Truth.

Health professionals can make a decent living off non-related causes and effects because people are simply too afraid to not believe them, for fear of getting worse—or dying. If a professional can convince the sufferer thoroughly enough that "their method" is the correct one, the professional might then help that person. But—once again—it only works if the person **deeply believes** in them, and in what they're advocating. Now the next question frequently asked is, "How do you know Dr. Sarno's success isn't from the same thing ... belief? Well, it is based on belief, the belief that you're physically okay.

With the information on TMS, countless people are healing from back pain; unlocking and unblocking everything that was preventing them from healing. They're casting off the chains their pain-practitioner had imprisoned them with, regarding the wrong causes and effects. However, Dr. Sarno's message is to stop doing ALL the interventionary measures. There is no ritual, no intervening, no intervener, nothing but learning. So what was it that fooled the person into healing? Nothing—except belief and the acceptance that unconscious emotions and conditioning patterns are the true sources of back pain.

## Placebo: Latin, *"I shall please"*

> *I've been invited to give a lecture at the 2004 North American Spine Society meeting in October, and that's going to be fun.*
> John E. Sarno, MD[5]

I tried all the spine techniques for aligning and realigning, and strengthening, and stretching. Those things all helped in the short run, but prolonged my pain in the long run. I've also seen hundreds of people who achieved temporary healing who were told they needed better posture, and a stronger core—but they didn't need those things. They needed to forget about those notions, and to focus on the need for their symptom. The problem with these therapeutic techniques is the same as the problem with injections, physical therapy, and surgery; and that problem is—they often work! Yes ... these treatments "can" work ... and sometimes do work. They work because of the most powerful healing phenomenon in all of medicine: **belief**—more commonly known in healing as **The Placebo.**

The placebo has received quite a bit of disparagement through the years as being a pejorative, with phrases like, "How do you know it wasn't just a placebo effect?" But a placebo isn't a bad thing. Who cares why the pain goes away? Pain is suffering, and suffering needs to end, right? Well, we know from experience that it may in fact matter how the pain goes away. I've seen people feel better after applying a magnet, or an ointment. When I talk to them about it being a placebo outcome, they say, "So what ... I don't care ... I feel better." What they don't know is that the problem remains, and could become serious. It's important how we take away our symptoms, or worse problems can be on the horizon. Covering melanoma with makeup doesn't mean it's gone.

Taking ulcer medicine doesn't solve the problem; it stops the symptom only, while the need for the ulcer may still be burning.

It should also be noted that placebos have saved the lives of many people. Belief can alter the physiology, moving the individual from ill to well. If the cause remains, though, the dis-"ease" may reenter by another means. If the placebo heals the sufferer, and the cause of the dis-ease does not remain, the individual will have been healed.

> *Most people spend more time and energy going around problems than in trying to solve them.*
>
> Henry Ford

There have been some amazing advances in techno-medicine that have saved millions of lives. Modern medicine is good. How and when it's used can be harmful. We need good doctors. This is not an anti-doctor message. This is an anti-status quo message. I'm referring to something called TMS, which everyone experiences in their lifetime.

For the most part, doctors and pain specialists are only mediators of health. They're trying their best, with what they have, are given, and what they know. They're constantly trying to administer any technique, pill, injection, surgery, or gimmick that will ease their patient's suffering. Due to techno-medicine, they've become like modern-day car mechanics, treating the human body like a mechanical chassis to be fixed, stabbed, drugged, strengthened, and straightened into good health. They're relying too much on drugs and procedures more and more, and less on their eyes and ears. However, the **person** is more than her structure; she's an emotional being. If she's not healing, then she's unconsciously blocking her healing for reasons that even she doesn't understand. The more prominent dilemma is that most healthcare providers appear to be driven to only treat symptoms. Ideally, the future doctor will use both: advanced techniques and mindbody techniques—which is currently called **Integrative Medicine**.

If a worker's ladder has a broken rung, and the worker continually falls off the ladder, continually breaking his leg, he can either keep putting a cast on his leg, or he can fix the ladder. Dr. Sarno fixed the ladder by discovering the Holy Grail for eliminating most suffering. He never had a method for treating back pain. He "cured it" by teaching sufferers how to understand the conflict that triggers the need for their pain.

*When people come to see me they are under the impression that their herniated disc is causing their pain, and I tell them "no it's not," (if I find that it's not) … the paradox is that, although they're well meaning, the doctors are contributing to the problem by attributing the pain to the wrong thing. So the patient has it in his mind that he's got a disc problem and that means the pain will NEVER go away. He has to be informed that the disc is NOT causing symptoms, and that the pressures in his life and the pressures that he puts on himself (are causing the problem), take note of that—that's the most important psychological phenomenon in this whole business. The pressure we put on ourselves to perform well, and to be good people, turns out to be very nice for society, but it turns out to generate a lot of internal anger—the unconscious mind wants none of this nonsense of having to be nice to people, and having to do the right thing.*

John E. Sarno, MD[19]

# 4

# The Tiger's Snare

## Examples: They're Grrreeeaatt!

We demand examples because examples prove to us that something is possible. We don't naturally accept something until we see it. There are literally tens of thousands of great examples of how the TMS process works. However, as I type this manuscript, I'm watching PGA golfer Tiger Woods, in Akron Ohio, withdraw from yet another golf tournament, due to back pain. My cell phone is also pinging with incoming texts, from golfing buddies, reminding me of the times I stated that his back surgery wouldn't work. But it gets more complicated than that, thus the continuing confusion. Here's a little more history for those who don't follow golf.

Tiger Woods had microdiscectomy back surgery in the spring of 2014, for what Tiger called "a pinched nerve." Five months after that surgery, on August 3, 2014, he withdrew from the WGC Bridgestone Invitational due to severe back spasms. He said he jarred his back jumping into a sand bunker. But from what I've experienced, the real reason Tiger went into severe back spasm today is that he suffers from TMS. The reason for his "new" pain today is that he never needed surgery; therefore, surgery never solved the problem as he thought it had.

Here's a bulleted history in order to draw a bigger picture for folks who may be curious:

- In 2004, Tiger had upper back pain and had to withdraw from the World Golf Championships-American Express Championship, on his way to Kilkenny, Ireland. He said that he hurt his back "sleeping awkwardly" on a jet (which is not possible).
  - ✓ **Going on in Tiger's life at the time:** Tiger was getting married in a few weeks, his father was dying, and he just lost his world #1 golf ranking for the first time. **Tension** was high—a diversion was needed.
- In May 2010, Tiger withdrew from The Players Championship with what he called a "bulging disc" in his neck, and tingling in his arm.
  - ✓ **Going on in Tiger's life:** His wife was about to serve divorce papers that week (shame from publicized personal events).

- In March 2014, Tiger fell prey to pain and withdrew from the WGC-Cadillac Championship.

  ✓ **Going on in Tiger's life:** Tiger was subpoenaed to testify in court the night before. The day after being subpoenaed he shot his worst round ever as a pro-golfer, at Trump-Doral. The next day, a Miami-Dade jury found Tiger Woods' company liable "for deceptive and unfair trade practices." The jury awarded $668,000 to the golf memorabilia retailer who had sued Tiger.

- Tiger had his first failed microdiscectomy surgery on March 31, 2014, and a second microdiscectomy on September 16, 2015, followed less than two months later by yet another procedure to relieve pain at the same site: a total of 3 procedures in an 18-month period.

  ✓ **Going on in Tiger's life:** He turned 40. Aging is one of the biggest triggers for TMS back pain because it reminds us that our clock is ticking, adding significant pressure to win faster, tick tick tick ....

> In almost every case, sufferers can trace their pain back to their life events: milestones of misery and happiness.

## Becoming Awake

Once people heal from their back pain they immediately begin to see TMS in everyone around them, as a new era dawns. The light of consciousness allows them to see what already exists. They begin to readily observe such types of life-event/pain correlations in their own lives, and in their loved ones. Here are a couple scenarios that I've personally witnessed:

- My friend's son joined the Army and was sent to Iraq on a tour of duty. My friend's knee suddenly began to hurt severely as soon as his son deployed. He believed, miraculously, that his knee had instantly gone bad, so he went to see his doctor. Routinely, and under the pressure to come up with an answer, his physician told him that he had a bad knee that needed to be scoped—cleaned out.

  ✓ **What really happened:** My friend's anxiety levels were sky-high when his son left. He complained to me often about his constant panic over his son's safety, and about his increased sleeplessness; he began taking anti-anxiety meds to block his emotional pain. His doctor was taught in medical school to find something—anything—when a patient comes into the office complaining of pain. The MRI showed microscopic tears and arthritis which are normal and incidental findings. His anxiety levels were causing his knee pain because of the unimaginable fear he had for his son's life. His brain was trying to help him cope by giving him a physical diversion. There was nothing wrong with his knee, so the surgery failed to bring relief.

> *What the MRI studies show in these people has nothing to do with the symptoms. And I have proven this concept ... they wouldn't get better if the structural abnormality were responsible for their symptoms.*
>
> John E. Sarno, MD[5]

- My former neighbor had severe neck pain. He went to a highly reputable pain clinic where he was told he had bulging/degenerated discs in his neck, and that they would need to insert a plate to relieve his pain. I pleaded with him not to have the surgery because there was nothing wrong with his neck. I told him that when it didn't work, his doctors would make up any excuse as to why it hadn't.

  ✓ **What really happened:** He was going through an extremely tense time in his life. He had the surgery and it failed. His surgeon then made the common statement when unnecessary surgery fails to bring relief: "We missed the spot we wanted to hit, we need to operate again." But he never needed surgery. His doctor was running him in circles chasing causes that didn't exist.

- A friend of mine, Hubert, who owned a restaurant, began having severe right shoulder pain. He went to his physician who told him he had tears in his rotator cuff and that he would need his shoulder scoped.

  ✓ **What really happened:** He was simultaneously opening a second restaurant under financial distress, and he was going through a rough divorce. The surgeon operated on his right shoulder and the pain shifted to his left shoulder. The surgeon then replied with yet another common and unfounded response: "Because of your right arm being in the sling, you've been using your left arm too much, placing too much strain on it ... we better go in and clean that shoulder out, too." The second surgery also failed to bring relief in that shoulder, naturally.

This appears to be exactly what Tiger Woods is experiencing now. The brain will shift the symptoms once the person believes the "original pain site" was somehow healed by the surgery (if the need for a diversion remains high enough). It often shifts the unpleasant sensations in a bilateral fashion from side to side, or even up and down. The objective of the brain is to continue to hide the rage over the unwanted self-imposed pressures and demands to be perfect: or in Tiger's case—purrrfect.

## Another Shoulder to Shoulder Example

> *Finally, it was recommended to me that I have surgery to fix the (shoulder) pain. After the surgery I developed the exact same pain in my right shoulder instead. I was also developing pains at this time in my low back and in my knee. I didn't understand what was going on, and so I continued to seek out help from a variety of conventional medical practitioners. It wasn't until a year ago that somebody told me about the concept of TMS which is put forth by Dr. Sarno. I read Dr. Sarno's books and they were a great help to me. Afterward though, I still had questions. Where do I go from here? Am I really able to recover? This is where Steve Ozanich's book, 'The Great Pain Deception; Faulty Medical Advice Is Making Us Worse' was absolutely an important part of my recovery ... Steve says in his book that no matter what a person's age is, no matter if they've had surgery, that they can heal and the pain can go away, if they want it to. I'm glad that this was also my experience. I no longer have chronic pain in my shoulders, in my back, in my knee, anywhere in my body. I can do 100% of what I was able to do before.*

Greg, "TMS Wall of Victory"

Everyone who has healed from TMS pain can see those around them making similar mistakes, focusing on their body's so-called flaws. It's only possible to see the mistakes made by others because of their own increased awareness, based on their own past mistakes. Those who have been through the experience are much happier and healthier because they know that the cure for chronic pain comes through self-education, not science.

> *I can't go back to yesterday because I was a different person then.*

Lewis Carroll, *Alice in Wonderland*

## The Golden Goose Laid an Egg

Tiger Woods is a living embodiment to the type of individual that experiences TMS, driven by self-imposed pressures, and seemingly impossible goals. His career goal has always been the same, to break

---

*Watch at YouTube "TMS Healing Wall of Victory - Testimonial Block #5 -
Dr. Chan and Greg"

Jack Nicklaus' records and to usurp Jack as the greatest golfer who has ever lived. Sheesh, is that all (I sayeth jokingly)? I don't think any of us can understand the demands he's placed on himself to accomplish such a feat. Adding to this tremendous pressure are the golf fans around the world "expecting" him to do it. He hears the clock in his head ticking, "You're getting older Tiger … hurry up!!"

I'm not judging Tiger by any means. He has made mistakes like all of us have, and I believe that deep inside he's a good person (there's that word "good" again). It's my personal opinion that his body is paying a price—but not for the demands he's making on his body; rather for the demands he's making on his emotional being. His doctors are sending him on wild-goose-chases by telling him that his healthy/strong body is somehow breaking (at the precise moments that his personal life is in upheaval and change). He does have a powerful mind, though, and at some point may attach himself to a placebo remedy, and temporarily heal—in that case, the true cause of his pains will remain forever unknown. However, Tiger should be aware: *Life will keep repeating itself until we finally pay attention.*

Some will ask, "Isn't it possible that Tiger has actually injured himself?" Yes, of course. Injuries do occur, but many TMS attacks look like real injuries. It's not likely that Tiger has injured his body during these precise times of personal turmoil, given his personality type, self-demands, correlated life-events, and common TMS symptoms. He's in better physical shape than any professional golfer in history, and TMS can be the most painful thing in clinical medicine. He not only has the perfectionistic personality, but he also has all the TMS signature hot spots: back pain, knee pain,* and heel pain. As each of his wounds heals, another steps up to the tee. This is the **Symptom Imperative** at work; a concept observed and conceptualized by some guy … oh yeah, Dr. Sarno!

- ❖ **Body symptoms are *changes*, such as:** swelling, stabbing, redness, weakness, itching, pins and needles, hot, cold, numbness, and pain.

- ❖ **Imperative *means*:** something that demands attention; required.

- ❖ **The Symptom Imperative *means*:** a physical change demanding attention. However, the thing demanding the attention is the person's psychic **conflict** and **needs**, not the body.

---

*Tiger once had a stress fracture in his tibia which is not TMS. But his brain may utilize that prior injury later if it wants to maintain a deception. It will remember the "old wound" if it needs to help him obsess on his body, when tension rises too high.

## "The Brain Will Not Be Denied"

Now let's look closer at the circus surrounding Tiger. Neither he nor his doctors appear to be placing enough emphasis on the obvious correlations between his symptoms and his life. They appear (at least publicly) to be chasing the medical industry's golden goose. So as Tiger withdrew from the WGC-Bridgestone golf tournament, he was still "TMSing." This means that his brain still needed to create a diversion to keep him unaware of the presence of surfacing emotions that his ego will not allow his conscious eye to see. They are repressed, so Tiger doesn't know they exist in him. He claimed as he left Firestone Country Club's parking lot that his new pain wasn't at the same location as the site of his recent surgery. Exactly!! With TMS, the brain will shift the pain to another area, often nearby, such as a spinal disc or two above, or below the old "injury" site.

This is Dr. Sarno's seminal observation of the Symptom Imperative. Whenever psychologically-induced pain is taken away by an artificial means like surgery, or drugs, or acupuncture, or manipulation, the brain will simply shift its focus somewhere else to keep the sufferer obsessed on something else, such as a new symptom or sensation, relocated pain, increased anxiety, sleeplessness, and oftentimes into severe depression. This occurs because the person has believed the recent healing procedure worked. But it didn't work, and the problem remains.

I've seen several people fall into clinical depression after what they believed was a successful surgery. They believed the surgery healed them—it had "pleased them"—and so their mind's eye imperatively* shifted to the true cause of their pain: the depression. Their pain had been serving as a diversionary channel for their depression all along by binding their fear to their body in order to keep them unaware of the extent of any darker thoughts. Once their brain had been pleased by the ritualistic technique of the surgery, and as long as their psychological conflict still existed, their brain sought out another specious focal point, shifting the symptom elsewhere. If the brain can't find a body problem that worries the sufferer enough to hold his attention, i.e., it isn't frightening enough, it often goes right to the source of the need for the diversion, the emotions: fear, isolation, and loneliness. This is very common after "artificial healing." The elimination of one symptom at the expense of another is not true healing.

**Artificial:** *imitation; simulated; sham.*

---

*Is anyone else impressed that I used the word "imperatively"? It's real, check it out.

Dr. Sarno frequently exclaimed, "The brain will NOT be denied!" You can run from your emotions but you can't hide from them. This is the "Tiger conundrum" that appears to be playing out repeatedly, and in countless others around the world. Surgery, drugs, injections, acupuncture, spinal manipulations and physical therapy are usually Band-Aids. They betray the sufferer by superficially covering the problem, creating even more confusion regarding what's really working, and what doesn't work. It's also embarrassing if you're on national television as the world watches you, like many pro-athletes, business leaders, professional actors, and anyone who places high standards on themselves to never fail. Observer eyes add even more pressure on the already *persecuted-Self*, and tension rises accordingly.

In a **Symptom Imperative shift** (SI-shift), the sufferer, like Tiger, now believes that his original back pain was indeed from a true spinal defect because that particular pain appears to be gone after surgery (or any therapeutic procedure). However, the problem is NOT gone. It has only changed form.

> *It just goes to show ya, it's always something, if it ain't one thing it's another.*
> Roseanne Roseannadanna, "Saturday Night Live"

This is a good time to make a couple important points.

❖ First: emotions are energy, and energy can never be destroyed,* it only changes form, thus the shifting.

❖ Second: emotions are hidden behind **the fear of the symptom**. If he doesn't fear his new pain, or new symptom, his brain will perpetually shift symptoms until it finds a place where he is worried about the new problem as being "real/structural/dangerous" … and if he fears this new symptom … there it will stay—exactly as his brain has designed. So the brain will create a physical sensation that feels like it's highly mechanical, or structural. It does this to make the sufferer think there's a body problem that needs to be repaired. The brain is quite creative in its desire to help, in a seemingly nefarious way.

Obsession is maintained behind the worry of the symptom, not just the symptom itself; worry subsequently magnifies it, determining its intensity, and longevity.

---

*The **law of conservation of energy** states that energy can neither be created nor destroyed, but can only change from one form to another form.

If she deeply integrates the concept of TMS, and no longer fears her "body symptoms," her brain will shift to something beyond body, such as hoarding, over-analyzing, confusion, pro-crastination, workaholism, extreme exercise, food paranoia, eating disorders, body dysmorphic disorder, or phobias, etc. This is the **Shadow Imperative**.

## Shadow Imperative

With the Shadow Imperative the brain has finally given up obsession on the body because the person no longer fears the physical symptoms. The helpful brain now takes aim at creating worry and obsession in the life of the person beyond the body's sensations—in its desperation to continue to divert fear. It's common for a sufferer to free himself of body-obsession worry, and then suddenly become afraid of something else. It also works the other way: such as, an alcoholic who stops drinking and then develops physical pain within days. The cause continues to seek resolution, in some form, because of the **Nature of Fear**.

 If the brain has something to say it will find a way.

## The Tiger's Blood

This is what I believe happened with Tiger Woods on August 3, 2014, in Akron, Ohio. The pressure he placed on himself to be perfect, to win, to be the best, to perform, and to never fail, became too much, once again. His anger and frustration needed yet another place to hide his sub-par performance. I watched him in Firestone's parking lot as I typed this section, holding his breath, grasping onto his vehicle for support, grimacing against wave after wave of searing disappointment. That's exactly how TMS manifests, and that's how I remember my own back pain, as waves of spasms cut through my overwhelming self-imposed demands.

Tiger's brain reduced bloodflow **as a favor** to him. It appears to be a classic case of TMS. And I thank Tiger for giving me a great example of how TMS works, just when I needed one. Now, of course, Tiger needs to be examined by a good Sarno-trained TMS physician like Paul Gwozdz, MD, in New Jersey, or Andrea Leonard-Segal, MD, in Washington, DC. The safety of the life is first, and foremost. I only mention Tiger because he was a purr-fect example today (sorry).

The more painful the back pain the more likely it's from TMS. And the more vociferously the sufferer rejects TMS as the cause of his pain, the more likely his pain is TMS—it's an indicator of how desperately he is hiding from his emotional truth.

Also, a delayed pain reaction is more likely TMS. If you lift something, or fall, and it doesn't begin to hurt until later, or keeps increasingly getting worse through the night, or during the week, it's more likely an emotional process.*

Certainly, anyone reading this book who has severe pain needs to be examined by a qualified MD to rule out danger. All I can say for certain is that Tiger Woods appears to be a typical TMS sufferer, with typical TMS symptoms, typical failed results, but an atypical bank account.

## The Symptom Imperative (SI): So Intuitive

The "snare" obviously applies to millions of people who are not a "Tiger." His example can be seen all around us. I told Dr. Sarno in April of 2012, that I felt the Symptom Imperative was his most insightful observation. He reconciled so many of our health problems with this particular observation. Long ago people would say, "That poor person is so unlucky in health!" They would have multiple surgeries, and an endless array of treatments in what seemed like health problem after health problem. We now know that the person has only one problem →TMS ... from self-imposed demands, driven by the ultimate fear of **separation/rejection**.

By ignoring our body's messages,† we set ourselves up for future health problems. If we properly address the root cause of pain and ill health, we solve most, if not all of our health problems. It's quite normal for a person to lose their lifetime of allergies once their back pain leaves. Some lose their food and pollen allergies, others have vision and skin improvement. The proper solving of the cause of back pain often allows other health problems to fade because the true problem was finally acknowledged, and dealt with.

---

*Watch at YouTube "TMS Healing Wall of Victory - Testimonial Block #8 – Heather"

†Ignoring the pain and ignoring the brain's message behind the pain are two very different things. Ignore the physical aspect of the pain, but try to understand why the pain has surfaced (what your deeper self is saying).

## The Last Stop

> *My life was filled with excruciating back pain and shoulder pain until I applied Dr. Sarno's principles, and in a matter of weeks my back pain disappeared. I never suffered a single symptom again ... I owe Dr. Sarno my life.*
>
> Howard Stern, DJ[20]

Dr. Sarno was the last stop for most of us sufferers, and yet, almost all the folks who he taught ended up healing. There were a small few who had serious psychological problems from childhood emotional abandonment that needed more care, and more support, in the form of psychotherapy.* As I mentioned above, the proof that herniated discs, spinal stenosis, and disc degeneration, et al., are not the causes of back pain, is that the sufferers heal, despite these so-called defects seen on the x-rays and MRIs. So it's impossible that those abnormalities were causing that specific pain.

As I also mentioned earlier, the **multidisciplinary approach** is the new in-vogue fashionable trend in healing back pain. But it's simply the medical industry approach repackaged to look different (insanity repeating itself). Every so often the names change to keep the industry thriving, and people confused, implying that the techniques, and healing know-how, have somehow advanced. But we have not gotten anywhere in pain healing; if we had, there would not be the many epidemics increasing in number all around us. It must be noted that medical science has learned a lot of fascinating pain stuff through new hypotheses such as Neuromatrix Theory—except for how to heal people, of course. Paradoxically, such theorizing is making people worse, because it's keeping us aimed at the physical aspects, and the searching leads us further from the resolution. The seeking of physical cures by peering deeper into the body serves to aid the brain in its great pain deception, and so the problems spread. *You can dissect a frog to see how it works, but you kill it in the process.*

## Clearing the Fog of Confusion

Here are two examples of how misconceptions compound the problem.

---

*Psychotherapy helps to better cope with the cause rather than internalizing it, which causes more pain. But it must be understood that psychotherapy will not work unless the sufferer understands what is occurring psychologically and physically. The pain will more often remain until the mindbody connection is made, despite working with a good psychotherapist.

- A mother is under overwhelming pressure at home and at work. She's imposing substantial demands on herself to take care of her children. She wants to be a great mother, employee, and wife. Her tension levels are high from her *desire to be perfect*. She bends to pick up someone's shoes and pain strikes in her low back. She goes to her chiropractor who tells her that she has slipped a disc. She believes her chiropractor because he or she has amazingly pinpointed the exact location of her pain, and because he or she wears a white coat (archetypal influence). The chiro sets up a series of spinal manipulations, tells her to rest, and over a few weeks she feels somewhat better. The chiro has saved her, she's appreciative, and brags to all her friends about how well spinal manipulation works.

  ✓ **What really happened:** She never slipped a disc because it's a physical/structural impossibility (without tearing apart the spinal structure). The chiropractor locates the exact location of her pain because that's where her brain has withdrawn the blood that created the knotted spasm. The area is seized, and locked up from a lack of oxygen, not a slipped disc. The spinal adjustment sessions simply diverted her mind's eye from her daily problems, providing yet another desperately needed distraction. She feels much better by the end of the sessions because her tension has faded. However, the true cause of her pain goes unrecognized, and she erroneously believes the adjustments worked. Later, due to the Symptom Imperative shift, her hip begins to lock up, and hurt. She heads back to the practitioner for more placebo treatments—the truth behind her pain is again buried in her body. She lives a life of on-and-off-again pain because she chases the wrong conclusions, adding to the slipped disc myth.

- A construction worker lifts a box and feels searing pain run through his back, and down the side of his leg. He goes to his doctor who orders an MRI. The MRI shows herniated discs at L3, L4, L5, and S1. What a shock! The worker is told that he needs to have those specific discs trimmed because they're pressing on his nerves. The worker has the surgery, and it goes well, "according to the surgeon." In a week or so, the construction worker is moving around much better, and his pain fades some. He tells all of his friends, "You should go see my surgeon, he's the best!" Months later, the worker's neck begins to hurt, or perhaps the spot right above or below the surgery site. He heads back to his surgeon for yet another disc trimming, and/or fusion.

✓ **What really happened**: The herniations in the worker's spine
were most likely there before he lifted the box, but there was no
reason to have an MRI beforehand. Most people have
herniations at these locations. However, his herniations have
nothing to do with his pain. His brain either randomly or
purposefully chose that particular spot. If the disc would have
been pinching his nerve he would have been paralyzed, the
nerve would have died quickly, and the dead nerve would no
longer have been able to send pain signals to his brain.
Therefore—if he had pinched a nerve, his pain would have
ended. What really happened is, when he lifted the box his brain
signaled for the bloodflow to be cut off because it was **ready** to
create a pain. All it needed was a trigger that the lifting
provided. The time away from his grinding job helped to lower
his tension level, along with the much needed downtime and
rest. His back pain was the message that he needed to slow his
life down, and that he needed some time away from his
responsibilities, which the surgery and the convalescence
provided. His sharp pain from lifting the box was only a trigger
that allowed him to force his mind onto his body and away from
the problems with his wife, kids, boss, or his last birthday when
he turned 30, 40, 50, or 60. The surgery was a red herring—
allowing (by forcing) him to rest. He draws the wrong
conclusions about his discs, back pain, and spinal surgery. And
his false assumptions continue ....

These weren't simply examples for explanatory purposes. They were
real-life situations that I witnessed. These two people healed
permanently after learning about TMS. This also holds true for
shoulder and knee surgeries, as well as hand and foot surgeries. Small
chronic partial tears are regularly blamed for causing pain in rotator
cuffs, as well as in knee menisci in knee pain. However, the TMS
healings prove that these aberrations were not causing pain—as with
spinal disc herniations—they're simply there. The brain will **sometimes
use those locations**[*] where the body has "changes," but once the
individual accepts TMS and takes the steps to heal, the pain leaves.

The medical industry is powerful in both its influence and its scope,
and disturbingly sufferers almost always desire quick medical fixes due
to their busy lives, as well as, the fervent desire to evade the true cause
of their pain.

---

[*]This is ranked #7 in the book, *Dr. John Sarno's Top 10 Healing Discoveries*

*The largest problem that we've had is that we present people
these options (healing back pain without surgery), and we're
excited about it, and people walk out and just want surgery.*

David Hanscom, MD, orthopedic surgeon,
who healed his own back pain with mindbody healing[21]

If a test is failed, it is either because of the teacher or the student,
or both. The word doctor from Latin, *docco*, means, "to teach." In the
case of most chronic pain, the teacher is teaching incorrect information
to the student, who is the sufferer, so of course the student fails. The
student relies on accurate information to pass the test. But the student
must also want to pass the test; must want to heal.

The probing question is, "Why do people let doctors perform
procedures on them that have little or no benefit?" The most obvious
answer is that they don't know they're being taught false things. But I've
also been told by sufferers, on numerous occasions, that they're afraid of
losing their doctor if they don't do everything he or she tells them to. But
it's even more complicated than that, and important to understand that
the better the doctor, the more that doctor will want you to get other
opinions, and will be more willing to work with you, not against you. A
doctor who demands that you do only what he or she wants, who won't
listen to your concerns, is a doctor who needs to be dropped.

What matters to you is what will please you—and what will
please you will heal you. Therefore, your opinion matters in
your health. Good doctors—a good person—will know that.

## Rising Misery and Ulterior Motives

There are hundreds of thousands of spinal fusion surgeries
performed every year in the United States alone. From 1998 to 2008
the number of fusions increased from 174,223 to 413,171[23]. The exact
number is not easy to find because neither the National Institutes of
Health nor the Center for Disease Control gathers those statistics. The
rate of spinal fusions was higher than all other inpatient procedures
between 1998 and 2008, making spinal fusion the second most
profitable surgery for hospitals behind heart surgery. From 2001 to
2011, the number of fusions increased 67 percent in Medicare patients
alone, despite the fact that there is no evidence to support that fusion
provides any benefits over spinal decompression surgery[22]. Thus,
surgeons were and (are) performing a more radically dangerous surgical
procedure, at an ever increasing rate of almost 70 percent that has zero
benefit over spinal decompression, which has almost no value itself.
Why do sufferers go through this risky process? Many are afraid to say

"no" to the physician because they're desperate for relief, and they want to believe that their health provider knows what he or she is doing. An underlying and unseen reason of course, is that the sufferers want to circumvent the real cause of the physical pain. What they appear to be looking for is a manner in which to cut the emotions out so they won't have to deal with them.

In November of 2013, Seattle orthopedic spine surgeon David Hanscom, MD, posed the question in his blog, "Am I Operating on Your Pain or Anxiety?" He writes, "It (surgery) rarely solves neck or back pain. It really doesn't work for anxiety. What relief are you asking your surgeon for?"[23].

In one of the greatest health books ever written, *The Will To Live; Your mind-Your health-and You*, Arnold Hutschnecker, MD, writes about this concept of cutting away emotional pain by surgically removing organs. "Sometimes an operation seems necessary for a sick person's emotional comfort, and sometimes we emerge from the hospital with some serious problem solved or some needed adjustment made. How much better, if we can, to attack the problem (emotions) and make the adjustment without sacrificing an organ in the struggle!"[24].

The end result is that we're receiving riskier, more expensive back pain procedures, with virtually no healing value beyond the sufferers' belief in the procedure. And, the problem grows ....

## Pointing Fingers

Critics have stated that TMS back pain is somehow "blaming the victim." But that's a lie, a purposeful untruth. There's no blame being cast on anyone, since the sufferer can in no way know he's doing it to himself. The process is completely unconscious, and is a true effort by the Self to survive. Would anyone blame a baby for crying?

❖ **It needs to be stated here:** This is not referring to acute injuries. An acute injury is an injury such as a broken bone, or a cut foot. Acute injuries repair quickly, and may need some repair from a medical procedure. The problem arises when the person lifts something, bends, or moves a certain way, triggering an acute pain attack, and thinks he has damaged himself, which then gets confirmed, incorrectly, by a pain practitioner. This is where the confusion lines up, and a domino effect of errors begins.

## Types of Pain

**Acute pain:** Occurs once, as a warning, a gift for survival. However, TMS can piggyback on an acute injury as a TMS opportunity. The confusion develops when the brain uses the acute injury, if it needs to at that time, in order to make the person believe the injury isn't healing. But it gets even more convoluted when TMS is triggered by a move or lift at which point the person thinks they have injured themselves, but the movement only triggered the TMS (Phase 2 TMS). There was no true injury; it just feels like it because it's so devastatingly painful.

Back pain can also suddenly appear without injury, while sleeping, or standing still, or sitting (Phase 1 TMS).

**Intermittent chronic pain:** Pain that occurs twice, or reoccurs only at certain times, such as times of day, seasons, family reunions, school, work, tax time, or holidays, etc. This type of pain is TMS, triggered by the event(s) through the senses, as a conditioned response (memory). When people have episodes of back pain they often feel that the pain returns due to an old injury, such as from an accident, or from lifting something many years ago (Phase 3 TMS). But as Dr. Sarno rightfully stated, "There's no such thing as recurrent pain from an old injury." The body healed completely, long ago. The brain only **uses the memory** of the old injury when it needs to hide guilt and shame, and divert awareness.

**Chronic pain:** Pain longer than a few months; this pain is a mindbody distraction. If enough time has gone by, beyond the point where the body "should have healed"—or, after it was repaired by a medical procedure—then the brain has covertly taken advantage of the opportunity, and is using the pain to provide a safe haven for hidden emotions. Acute injuries that blend into chronic injuries are driven by unconscious emotions and memory. Pain does not last a lifetime without emotional/conditioning involvement.

Now if a joint, such as a knee, or shoulder, has structurally worn out then it will need to be replaced by a medical procedure. The tragedy is that replacements are being done every day on healthy joints that the brain is only using as a diversion. The doctors and patients don't know about Tension Myoneural Syndrome (also referred to as The Mindbody Syndrome), and so any type of normal changes to the joint, as in wearing and tearing, get wrongly blamed for the pain.

# 5

# Studies: Sources of Confusion

*Always learning but never able to come to a knowledge of the truth.*

2 Timothy 3:7

Every day, I read about experts describing worthless health studies.* I subscribe to daily Google watch lists for health and pain studies, and the information is meaningless hogwash, more often than not. A couple that come quickly to mind are studies claiming that having pronated feet causes low back pain, and that back pain "is linked to obesity." Obese people are often depressed people. Linking pronated feet and obesity to back pain is like linking car crashes to wearing seat belts. Most people in car crashes are wearing seat belts. So seatbelts must be a cause of the crash. It's ludicrous—but people loooove numbers. Numbers are their obsessive diversion.

Billions are spent every year to produce worthless causes and effects that are called: **scientific evidence**. Just because a study yields "a result" does not mean the result is true. In fact, the results are more likely to be untrue, depending on a mixture of biases and prejudices. According to John Ioannidis, Professor of Health Research and Policy at Stanford School of Medicine, "Most research findings are false for most research designs and for most fields."[25]

Ioannidis' studies on studies reveal that more than half of published research findings are false (less likely to be true) because of many factors, such as financial interests, power of the study, bias, effect size, prejudice, inability to replicate the original findings, and "when more teams are involved in a scientific field in chase of statistical significance."

---

*Science is good. Almost everything we have both good and bad, came from learning, driven by imagination and the quest to understand. However, the problems in seeking meaningful answers come from manipulated information, studying just to get published, and meaningless cause and effect results from those with vested interest in certain outcomes.

> *There is increasing concern that most current published research findings are false ... Simulations show that for most study designs and settings, it is more likely for a research claim to be false than true. Moreover, for many current scientific fields, claimed research findings may often be simply accurate measures of the prevailing bias ... There is increasing concern that in modern research, false findings may be the majority or even the **vast majority of** published research **claims**. However, this should not be surprising. It can be proven that most claimed research findings are false.*
>
> John P. A. Ioannidis

We persistently attempt to step closer, hoping to see better, but sometimes we need to step back to distance ourselves from the details to view the entire picture. Too often, lost in the business of studying health, and in making false claims, is healing.

At the time of this writing, a Northwestern University Feinberg School of Medicine[26] study hit the AP circuit claiming that smokers are three times more likely than nonsmokers to develop chronic back pain. Scientists studied the nucleus accumbens and medial prefrontal cortex circuits of the brain, and had observed that people who had a strong connection between these "two parts" were more likely to develop chronic pain—and that smokers had a very strong connection between these two parts. They claimed that once the smokers quit smoking, the activity in these areas dropped dramatically. However, the activity in these areas could have dropped dramatically for an infinite number of other reasons.

This particular study claims to be the first research to link smoking to chronic back pain. However, the designers didn't consider that the smokers also may have felt better about themselves after stopping smoking, and may have been in a better emotional state, and decided to renew their lives with hope, which could also have lowered the activity in these two areas. We can never know because studies can't measure the person, the motivations, and those pesky emotions.

The study's designers stated that smoking didn't cause back pain, but made it worse by making the person "less resilient" to pain. But everyone that I've ever met, have known, and have worked with, had their back pain increase dramatically after they stopped smoking because they lost their anxiety soother, and the distraction ritual that smoking provided them.

Anxiety often necessitates the diversion of back pain, and smokers are generally more anxious people. There are numerous reasons that a person's brain will have lowered activity between the nucleus accumbens and medial prefrontal cortex circuits of the brain; but studies don't consider anything other than the current hypotheses (null and alternative).

# GIGO: Garbage in, Garbage out

> *You can come up with statistics to prove anything, forty percent of all people know that.*
>
> Homer Simpson, "Homer the Vigilante"

I've done several shows where the producer wanted me to "bring my studies." Why would I bring something that has no value? Why would a kamikaze pilot wear a helmet? Why does a psychic need to ask me for my credit card number? Why is a round pizza put into a square box and cut into triangular pieces? Why is the word abbreviated so long? Many things don't make sense, and studies are at the top of the list.

Studies can offer a useless conclusion resulting from:

- The spurious correlation (false connection);
- The desire to simply support a predetermined position;
- The need to spend all the grant money.

As with high-tech imagings, studies can add greatly to the perplexity of events by assigning false meaning to unrelated relationships. However, many people live and die by numbers. Regrettably, I've resorted to using studies to support my own positions against the value of studies' usefulness. But when you're trying to make a point to someone it's best to use the language they speak. Studies aren't a bad process; we need to learn somehow. The problem often is one of how the study is set up. If it's set up poorly, or is weak to begin with, the results will be worthless; but their worthlessness doesn't stop people from citing them if they need to. Every day it's evident that people accept valueless study results with common discussion-starters like, "A recent study claims ...."

> *Statistics are used much like a drunk uses a lamppost: for support, not illumination.*
>
> Vin Scully, sportscaster

Many depend on inanimate numbers to tell them if they will heal, or even live; their lives are guided by their belief in inorganic characters. But many of the numbers resulting from the many studies are a large part of the confusion because they're often mixed and matched to form a brilliant prosaic of nothingness. The reason is: **correlation does not imply causation**.

Because you got this from that doesn't mean that this was caused by that (not from Dr. Seuss).

For example, past studies have indicated that tea may prevent lung cancer, over coffee. But it happens that tea drinkers rarely smoke compared to coffee drinkers. So of course they have fewer incidents of lung disease, duh. In spurious correlations, there's always a third factor in play that the study's designers haven't taken into consideration, or don't care to observe. Or there's simply a rush to tie factors together, like seeing the ground wet and claiming that wet ground causes rain. This is seen in the assumption that herniated discs, disc degeneration, and spinal stenosis cause back pain. They do not. The unknown third factor in the disc-pain-herniation *correlation error* is the reduced oxygen flow via the autonomic nervous system, from tension.

Andrew Weil, MD, describes listening to a lecturer at the North American Academy of Musculoskeletal Pain at which Weil was the keynote speaker. The lecturer described the current data on the lack of correlation between back pain and the abnormalities as seen on MRIs and x-rays. Weil states, "He (a speaker) showed x-rays and scans of patients that looked so awful you could not believe these people could stand or walk, yet they were free of pain and had normal mobility. In other cases, people were immobilized by pain, yet their spines looked normal. To my mind, all of this information was consistent with Dr. Sarno's philosophy[27]."

## Study This!

On July 14, 1994, Maureen Jensen and her colleagues published their findings in the New England Journal of Medicine on the lack of correlation between spinal disc bulges and pain. They examined 98 people who had never had back pain and found that 64 percent of them had disc abnormalities. Other similar studies have shown the same results: back pain has little or no relation to disc bulges. Why doesn't anyone worship those numbers? Many sufferers only see studies as valid if they show that the body is at fault. Those that show the body is not failing tend to be ignored.

*In 2004 (after decades of pain), I read a book by Dr. Sarno, I began to follow his regimen, I haven't had a back pain since, why isn't THIS being looked at?*

Senator Tom Harkin of Iowa[28]

Former Iowa Senator Tom Harkin healed from decades of debilitating back pain after he discovered Dr. Sarno's work. I'll never forget the scene in the Senate building where he convened a meeting on "Pain in America." The panel was filled with medical scientists, and a pain sufferer, who had all brought their numbers, except for Dr. Sarno. None on the panel had read Dr. Sarno's work, who sat quietly at the end of the panel. None of them knew that he had already discovered the cause and solution to most of what they were there for, but none seemed interested. They were intent on delivering their numbers to the Senate panel. At one point in the meeting Senator Harkin told his story of trying everything, and then finding Dr. Sarno's work and healing. He then raised Dr. Sarno's books in the air and asked the panel guests, "Why isn't this being looked into?" The blank stares on their faces make my position in this book stronger. They just weren't that interested in success. They were focused on the science; inanimate veneration.

*There is lots of research (on mindbody healing). It's published in bona-fide and major medical journals, but it disappears without a trace. It's like it has no impact on practice. It's DESPITE the evidence, not for the lack of it, that we practice the way we do.*

Gabor Mate, MD[12]

Scottish philosopher David Hume had long proclaimed that causation could never be proven, and philosopher of science Karl Popper firmly maintained that it's impossible to prove a relationship, only to disprove it. It could easily be proven that herniated discs don't cause back pain by actually looking at all the people who heal from it, but who still have those same spinal abnormalities.

## Set up the study:

**H₀ (null hypothesis):** Herniated discs cause back pain

**Hₐ (alternative hypothesis):** Herniated discs do not cause back pain

It would be fairly simple to disprove the null hypothesis and to prove the alternative hypothesis, by grabbing the first person off the street with back pain, showing him the information on TMS and watching him heal. This happens often.

The alternative hypothesis could then be reinforced by grabbing the next 100 people off the street with herniated discs, and back pain, showing them the information on TMS, and watching them heal. This would be relatively simple except for one thing: those people would have to **believe and accept TMS**. Belief is the unknown variable in most health studies, and the reason that so many experiments have small value. In studies involving people, and health, you can't measure intent, love, fear, need, desire, motivation, or belief: effects of emotions.

For psychological and sociological reasons, we've bought into the notion that spinal disc bulges cause pain, and that truth can only be identified within a clinical trial. I realize that some studies have some merit and value. But a number from a study doesn't necessarily solve a problem, or get us any nearer to the truth. Fire can't be extinguished with fire. Is the zebra white with black stripes, or black with white stripes? The answer is … who cares? Just enjoy the zebra.

> *One of the most untruthful things possible, you know, is a collection of facts, because they can be made to appear so many different ways.*
> Karl A. Menninger, MD, founder of the Menninger Clinic

## Thinking Versus Feeling

The late, great, psychiatrist Carl Jung observed that **intellect** and **feeling** were polar opposite functions, noting that "nothing inhibited feeling like thinking." Pain sufferers often tend to be intellects, in the sense that they use thinking as their coping mechanism, and ignore their feeling, which would be their inferior function if thinking is their superior function. People often demand science and numbers as part of their intellectual barrier, as a defense against feeling. They trust their head, not their heart. "The thinker" represses her feelings strongly, resisting their integration into consciousness, and relies primarily on thinking for survival. In this way she protects her heart from emotional pain.

> *The inferior function is practically identical with the dark side of the human personality.*
> CG Jung, MD[29]

At one point in their lives, the thinker-analyzers were hurt deeply as children; so much so, that they ablated their darker shameful feelings in order to hide them, to not get hurt anymore, subjugating their feelings to thinking. As adults, they live in their heads to avoid further emotional pain, using thinking as their primary means of coping, never aware that they possess an emotional blind spot (until pain strikes). The reason they use thinking is that they have little control over their emotions; they're overwhelmed by them, and so the emotions are simply avoided (repressed). The thinker-analyzers aren't even aware that they're not feeling certain emotions because thinking has become their modus operandi for dealing with life's problems. They rationalize rather than feeling, and reject truths that aren't "supported by facts." But as emotional beings, the emotions are ever present even when unrecognized.

**Ablate:** *made less in size or amount or degree.*

TMS naysayers and skeptics demand science and numbers as proof of what is already true. Thinking has become their way of TMSing, of avoiding certain aspects of their lives that are too emotionally painful. So it's natural that they would demand science as a way to avoid healing. Numbers can't hurt them, unless they accept the numbers as true and then assign a feeling to them.

## Works for A. Weil

I admire integrative medicine pioneer Andrew Weil, MD, for his courage of conviction in healing. He has said that he had to go with what was working in his patients, not what the studies were saying. "What works" is often what the patient believes will work, if it pleases him. And so his symptoms may be relieved through the ritual of the "act of administering a process." However, the relief of his symptoms doesn't necessarily mean that he is "healed." It just means that his brain believed the act helped him. True healing is a much deeper process that seeks resolution of conflict, since most **chronic pain is a defense against truth.** Truth doesn't need to be searched for, it just needs to be allowed because it already is. Just as Dr. Sarno didn't need studies to prove that people were healing by the masses; they already were.

There are studies and beliefs popping up constantly that contradict previous notions, depending on many factors, such as who paid for the study and what the sample size was. More meaningful numbers come from watching the trends across many studies, known as **meta-analysis**: aka, research on research. But for certain, what once was, may not now be, as the conscious waters shift with the prevailing tide.

- Milk: Once thought to be the best thing for us. Then became the scourge to be avoided. Now, good again.

- Leeches: Once used for health rituals, then considered a joke. Now beneficial again.

- The appendix: Prophylactic appendectomies once routinely performed. Now many scientists feel the appendix may have an immune system responsibility.

- Tonsils: Tonsillectomies once routine events, now rarely done.

- PSA: Blood PSA levels were once considered the standard care for preventing prostate cancer, now the consensus is turning toward the finding that it's a fairly useless number.

- The advice on avoiding hurting the back, by bending the knees and keeping the back straight while lifting is deeply ingrained in the public consciousness as the "correct way to lift." But now, researchers at Aberdeen University say that the way we should lift actually depends on the shape of our spine.* Therefore, not everyone should lift the same way!

The main point is NOT that the studies consistently contradict each other and waste money, which they often do; the point is that the studies' numbers can be meaningless unless the people accept the results to be true. This falls under the **Nature of Truth,** which tends to shift with the sweeping winds.

 Which determines Truth: studies ... or beliefs?

Many notions currently accepted as true ... are not true:

- Ostriches don't stick their heads in the sand.
- The Earth spinning around really fast doesn't keep us from falling off by "pulling us down." The Earth curves space-time around us and pushes us down to Earth (Einstein's Theory of General Relativity, 1915).
- Lightning can strike the same place repeatedly.
- Bats are not blind.
- Chameleons don't change colors to blend into their surroundings; their colors change according to mood, or to communicate.
- Lemmings do not engage in mass suicide.
- White is not a lack of color, it's every color combined.
- Mount Everest is not the tallest mountain on Earth (base to summit).
- Pandora's Box is not a box, it's a jar.
- A mother bird does not abandon the baby birds if you touch them.
- Different sections of the tongue are not responsible for different tastes[30].
- Humans have many more than five senses, including temperature sensing, kinesthetic sense, balance, and nociception (the ability of a body to sense potential harm; *à la* pain).
- Polar bears don't have white fur, they have clear fur and black skin[31].

---

*The conclusion in the summary of the study stated that individuals with straight spines squatted to lift while those with curvy spines stooped, indicating that the way we move to pick up a load is associated with the shape of our spine[82]. None of this is relevant to pain, of course. Study on ....

- Egg yolks do not raise blood cholesterol levels. Saturated fat (palmitoleic acid) intake that is doubled and tripled does not drive up the level of saturated fat in a person's blood; carbohydrates do[32]. The level of saturated fats in the system is determined by carbs, meaning that the level of harmful saturated fats in the diet comes primarily from carbohydrates, not those evil eggs, butter, bacon, ice cream, and red meats, etc.

The main source of the harmfully bad fats in the diet that are causing the major health and heart problems come from the white breads, pastries, sodas, and other highly processed or refined foods.

> *There is widespread misunderstanding about saturated fat. In population studies, there's clearly no association of dietary saturated fat and heart disease, yet dietary guidelines continue to advocate restriction of saturated fat. That's not scientific and not smart.*
>
> Jeff Volek, PhD, The Ohio State University

- Etc.ɔtᴲ ... may be reversed in the future at some point!

Certainly, one day the public will collectively and consciously accept (as truth) that the ritual of trimming spinal discs was a huge medical mistake, in the vast majority of cases. The thinking is already reversing on many modern techniques. However, it's still important to ask, "Does the human body ever need to be scientifically repaired from the outside?" The answer is always yes, of course. Modern medical transplants and grafting have facilitated some life-altering miracles. A diseased or very old worn joint may need to be scientifically upgraded. There are also some really odd spinal situations where the back may need to be repaired by a surgical procedure. But the chance of anyone who is reading this being in that category is nearly zero.

The key for the future doctor is in balancing when the medical engineering is actually hurting the patient by covering over the cause of the symptom: placating the deeper desire of avoidance; and then of course, finding a doctor who cares if she or he is doing more harm. This may be the tougher task. With great power comes greater responsibility, and those who have influence over our health need to care more about the patient than the procedure.

> *From everyone who has been given much, much will be demanded; and from the one who has been entrusted with much, much more will be asked.*
>
> Luke 12:48

## Subsets of Truth—
## Assigning Numbers to the Unquantifiable

*A number is an infinitesimal piece of Truth—incrementally chasing Truth, never revealing it.*

It dawned on me one day while I was looking at a new study published in JAMA regarding the great value of acupuncture. I kept all documents during my research for future support (CYA). So I dug into my pile of papers and found a report from the same prestigious medical journal talking about how acupuncture was worthless. I laid them out, side by side and read them as they summarily contradicted one another. One study said acupuncture was great! The other said it didn't work. And to solidify the point, during the writing of this book, yet another study was published in JAMA on Sept. 30th, 2014, called "Acupuncture for Chronic Knee Pain," proving that acupuncture for chronic knee pain is worthless. Yet people still want to believe in acupuncture because acupuncture pleases them.

Neither laser nor needle acupuncture conferred benefit over sham for pain or function. Our findings do not support acupuncture for these (knee pain) patients[33].

As could be predicted, then arose the fiery formation of impassioned people complaining about how the Hinman study was wrong, and how acupuncture stopped their knee pain. But what they aren't aware of is their own power of belief.

It's obvious that cause and effect can be measured with great accuracy, but what do all the contradictory numbers tell us about the person, and why she is in pain? Religious studies scholar, Houston Smith, phrased it perceptively: "Meaning slips through the instruments of science as the sea slips through the nets of the fisherman." An extraordinarily large number of pain sufferers who contact me have recently had a loved one die. Science doesn't consider those sorts of things, nor can it measure the impact that emotions and separation have on pain.

Not only do studies often contradict one another (especially in the earlier replications of the original findings),* they also become limiters for many people. I've seen **numbers harm people** by telling them that successes are not possible. Not only have I seen it, I was one of those

---

*This is the **Proteus phenomenon**. Many studies that follow an initial study's findings tend to contradict the original study's findings due to *publication bias*. The researchers are prejudiced against the original study's results, so they set out to prove it wrong with selective and distorted reporting, and by manipulating the analysis.

harmed. If the numbers aren't good, the sufferers' beliefs begin to match the negative numbers, altering, stagnating, and guiding their biology toward the worst possible outcome.

## The Two Percent Solution

In 1987, Dr. Sarno conducted a random follow-up survey of 109 of his patients whose pain was originally attributed to a herniated disc. He diagnosed each of them as having TMS and they all went through his healing program. The follow-up showed that 88 percent were healed, 11 percent were much better with some restricted activity, and 2 percent were unchanged. In the past 16 years that I've been working with TMS and consulting, almost every single sufferer has felt they were part of the two percent who may not heal—because of Dr. Sarno's follow-up study's numbers. Sufferers glue themselves to what may not be possible, rather than freeing themselves to what is possible. The two percent "negative" number becomes an anchor around their necks, their new obsession, preventing them from moving forward. **Their confidence was limited by the numbers.** I, too, thought that I would be one of the two percent who could never heal because the tendency of a negative perfectionist is to look at the impossibility, and to make that their probability. In such cases, the studies hinder healing because people believe numbers are true, so they latch onto things like surveys, and what other people are doing, or not doing.

Belief is THE master key to healing—belief that you WILL heal.

## The TMS Skeptic: Shoot First Ask Questions Later

I hear it frequently from skeptics (defeatists), regarding back pain, "You're wrong, my back is a mess!!"... or ... "You're wrong, my doctor told me I have a bad back!!!"... and ... "Where are your numbers??" It's extremely difficult to do a mindbody study because most people won't volunteer. Who wants to have their back cut open, only to hear later, "Ha ha ... you were fooled!" In addition, the numbers are unstable and highly subjective because healing is a feeling that is almost impossible to assign a value to.

For example, I used to ask sufferers to rate their healing progress on a scale of 1-10. Some have said that they felt much, much, much better; their pain was a level 10 before they found my book, and weeks later they now feel they're at a level 4. They're happy again and doing whatever they want without worries; they are living, laughing, and loving life. They feel whole again, and at greater peace.

Others have told me that they were once at a level 10, then found out about TMS, and are now quickly at a level 3, but they still fear their pain, and tell me they "have a long way to go." Hence, one has numerically gauged her healing as less … but feels great, and has no fear, or restrictions. The other has gauged her healing as numerically better than the other sufferer, but has self-restrictions, with lingering worry and fear. So what good are those numbers? And what about people who heal after the study is over? Healing can take place at any time, and trying to heal within a specific timeframe further inhibits healing.

 Mindbody studies are **subjective** in nature because people view challenges and improvement differently, through different perspectives.

The only numbers that have meaning are those that include the guy over there playing with his kids again, or the woman hiking and laughing again, and the teenager smiling again. My definition of being healed is the point at which you're happy again, and re-engaged in life, without fear.

## Naysayers Pounding Defenseless Scarecrows

 *There are two objectionable types of believers: those who believe the incredible and those who believe that belief must be discarded and replaced by the scientific method.*
Max Born, quantum physicist

The extremely high rate of TMS healings isn't persuasive enough for many folks because healing comes in a different manner than they expected. One of the most common rejections of TMS is, "This stuff is just a bunch of anecdotal stories." Hearing about people healing from pain at the highest rate of success doesn't mean anything to them; they demand science as proof, wrapped in numbers. Do we need science to prove that birds can fly? Skeptics hold tight to their personal agony by hiding behind claims such as a "lack of science," as a psychological defense mechanism. Common defenses against healing include:[*]

- Science doesn't support it!

- Everyone is different, what works for one person may not work for another.

---

[*]List regenerated from the book *Dr. John Sarno's Top 10 Healing Discoveries*

- Dr. Sarno's work is okay, but it didn't work for me.
- Anger didn't make my back disc herniate!
- TMS is stupid, my body makes noises!
- My pain is real!!!
- I was in an accident. No one is going to tell me my pain is all in my head!!
- Dr. Sarno doesn't know what pain is or he would never say such things!

These common themes of attacks against TMS healing are **straw men arguments**,* proclaimed in order to defend pain, so that the real cause can remain hidden (#2 in Dr. Sarno's most salient discoveries). More important, none of these statements is true. A straw man argument is a method to "try to" discredit an opponent through creating an illusion of defeating his position, by replacing his proposition with a false proposition (the straw man), and then knocking down the "straw man," instead of the original proposition. Victory is then claimed. But in the straw man case, the antagonist **misrepresents the original position**, and so the only thing that is successfully refuted, or struck down, is the false argument—not the original position. The straw man technique is employed because it's much easier to knock down a false proposition than a true proposition. For a straw man argument to be successful, *it must rely on the audience being uninformed.* Here's how it works:

> **Observer:** Proclaims proposition X
> **Antagonist:** Makes up a false proposition Y, and then argues against proposition Y instead of X. In defeating Y, claims victory against X.

### Example 1:

> **Dr. Sarno:** Herniated discs don't cause back pain.
> **Skeptic:** Anger didn't make my back disc herniate!

Since herniated discs don't cause back pain, the skeptic builds a straw man argument to knock down the good doctor's work. Here, the naysayer makes a passing reference to something about anger causing discs to herniate. In his mind, he has successfully defeated the TMS position by knocking down his own claim.

---

*In England the straw man is referred to as an Aunt Sally.

### Example 2:

**Dr. Sarno:** *This (back snapping sound) is a common description of onset and invariably suggests to patients that something terrible has happened to their back, though we know in retrospect that this is not the case.*

**Skeptic:** TMS is stoopid, my body makes noises!

Since noises can't cause pain, the skeptic has set up a straw argument to prevent his own healing. The extrapolation can continue for all the other arguments, such as, "Dr. Sarno doesn't know what pain is." Because he in fact suffered greatly from his own back pain and various other severe symptoms, the naysayer's statement disproves nothing. And the argument of, "My pain is real" can't stand on its own either because Dr. Sarno stated, "It (TMS) could produce more pain than anything I've ever seen in clinical medicine." Since he proclaimed TMS to be the most painful thing he had ever seen, the argument of pain "being real" can't successfully refute the original proposition, which in this case is already about real pain.

Other defense mechanisms need to be taken one at a time, such as, "I tried Dr. Sarno's quackery but it didn't work!!" This is a deep misunderstanding. It simply doesn't happen that way. You have to have full belief in the TMS process or it doesn't work. You can't have doubt, and cynicism, and ulterior motives, and still expect to heal. So it's a straw man claim to have "tried the quackery" and had it fail. The desire to heal is a full commitment process that takes a lot of deep introspection, time, hard work, and **belief**. Healing requires a deep desire to heal, not just to get rid of pain. It took me almost 2 years to heal from 30 years of back pain. Anyone claiming to have read the book and then stating that "it didn't work for me" doesn't understand the message. Sadly, they then try to steer others away from a process that could help them heal. What kind of a person would do such a thing? Who would thwart the most successful healing message in history? Why would anyone want to bring down a message that consistently helps others? The answer lies with the cause of most of our other life problems, within ego.

## The Controlling Ego

Skeptics often resort to **The Argument of Incredulity** to defend their position. This tactic is used when the arguer decides that something is not possible because he can't understand it. It's incredulous to him so he feels it can't be true. He then argues with his own inability to understand as "proof" that the notion can't possibly be true. Simply put, if he can't understand it, that's his proof that it's not true. And yet back pain is being healed virtually every day with TMS understanding.

If you read through the one-star reviews at Amazon for *Healing Back Pain*, it's clear that not one of those reviewers understood the message. Each thought they had grasped the concept and then attempted to refute it using a punch drunk scarecrow that's been knocked down so many times it has trouble standing. The naysayers hear part of the message, and draw an entire universe of wrong conclusions. A large culprit in the skeptical misunderstandings is the wild-west Internet where anyone can say anything, about anybody—true or untrue.

I rarely read book reviews but for the purpose of this book I read some of the one-star reviews trashing *Healing Back Pain*. On one review, I noted that the reviewer was an Amazon power reviewer[34] who posted nearly 3000 reviews. But in his review of *Healing Back Pain* he didn't say one thing that was true about Dr. Sarno's book. So I contacted him to tell him that what he wrote was false. He responded to me in the comments by telling me he hadn't read it. He said that he flipped randomly to several pages and it made his back hurt.

So the reviewer never read the book but gave it a terrible review for being a bad book. This is the attitude those of us who have healed, and who are trying to help, face on a daily basis. The rejecters don't read it, or only read parts and don't quite understand it, then condemn it so that no one else can gain benefit from it. It's much like the military strategy of *scorched earth*. If they can't understand it they want to make sure no one else can utilize it to get rid of their suffering. It is an extremely egocentric attitude. This point is critical to understand in healing. Ego is the very thing that causes our suffering because it blocks the truth behind our suffering by shielding full consciousness. When we reject the very thing that can take our suffering away we must pause, and ask "why?" Why did I throw *Healing Back Pain* across my room? Why do so many others refuse to see the solution to their problems? The answer is that, if we accept that our spine is okay and healthy we must then accept responsibility for our lives. If we blame our body for our problems we never have to admit that things haven't gone the way we wanted. It's not our fault we just got unlucky with a bad spine. Of course physicians help us in the decoy by falsely claiming that we have defective spines.

The back pain is holding us accountable for what we refuse to accept as true. Hence the true cause of back pain must be strongly rejected. But remember, everyone will come to truth when they are ready. The only difference between those who have accepted TMS and healed and those who haven't is that those who have healed were **finally ready** to give up their suffering.

**Accountable:** *Responsible, answerable, subject to the obligation to report, explain, or justify something.*

Other such defenses against healing, like, "I was in an accident. No one is going to tell me my pain is all in my head!!" are the reason that the straw man argument is also referred to as "attacking what the other person never said." No one has ever stated that back pain is imagined, or all in the head. TMS is also not about injuries; no one has ever said that it was. The only way the straw argument even works is if the people observing the argument are wholly uninformed, which most are. The bystander then sees the argument and feels as though the skeptics make a good point. But the naysayers have only refuted comments that were never said, or even implied.

Ego—the emotional component of mind—can be very controlling when it desires to block full awareness.

It's important for the frustrated messengers of TMS to remember the Deepak Chopra statement that, "People are doing the best they can from their own level of consciousness." When someone gets angry at something they don't understand, the person who does understand should react with some compassion, not equal anger. However, due to the naysayer's impassioned backlash, most people who have healed from back pain simply stay silent. They want to help, but they don't want to deal with the combativeness.

Anyone can jump on the Internet to see the massive numbers of people who have healed from back pain, thanks to Dr. Sarno, and who are now happy—and are trying to help others. One group accepts TMS and is happy. The other group angrily rejects TMS, continues to suffer, and tries to prevent others from benefiting from the message. The aphorism clearly describes that, "Pain is inevitable but suffering is a choice."

# 6

# The EPS Dénouement

## The Unmuddling of:
## Ego, Placebo, and Symptom Imperative

The confusion and all the resultant failures regarding the true cause of back pain can be illuminated through the deeper understanding of the complex combination of three elements:

- **E**go
- **P**lacebo
- **S**ymptom Imperative

> **Dénouement:** *the resolution and final climax, as all the confusing pieces are suddenly tied together for clarification.*

If you're in pain, you can heal, by understanding, not by doing. You will need to open your mind to something that you may think is incredulous, even impossible. I thought it was absurd when I first heard about TMS, so I rejected it outright. My **ego** wouldn't allow for the truth within me to rise to consciousness, and the consistent **placebo** treatments were pleasing me with intermittent relief from pain, while the **Symptom Imperative** was ever present and shifting—fooling me into thinking I had been helped with my last treatment.

Whether it was manipulations, spinal strengthening, spinal aligning, hanging upside down, steroidal injections, or acupuncture, etc.—I tried them all; but none worked in the long run. Once I realized that my ego had been shielding me from certain aspects of myself (aided by continual incorrect diagnoses), I began to look deeper into TMS, and I began to heal—deeply, and permanently. But I had to first:

- **Admit** that my ego wouldn't accept that my back was okay;
- **Realize** that placebos were only pleasing me;
- **Learn** that medical procedures were keeping me in pain by allowing me to further avoid the cause, as each sham procedure forced a new symptom shift.

## Ego: The Destructive Force of "Me"

*The hard core of egotism is difficult to dislodge, except rudely.*
Paramahansa Yogananda, *Autobiography of a Yogi*

Ego is Latin for, "I," e.g., different, or separately unique. There has been much written on ego, with many different opinions, usages, and definitions, but it is not necessary to discuss it all here. It gets complicated, and is mostly irrelevant. We are only concerned with how ego relates to healing, or more particularly, to protecting suffering and *not* healing.

Ego aids in suffering when the person says: "I" won't consider anything other than what "I" believe; "I" don't believe my emotions are causing my pain; "my" back pain is unique—different—from all the other sufferers' pain. However this was one of Dr. Sarno's most excellent discoveries of observation. The brain creates a real physical terror of such frightening sensation that the unaware sufferer will think his pain is damaging his body; his brain is hoping to create fear and worry. On the outside the suffering individual is normally calm and quiet in appearance, a superego state— at the direction of ego. *I can't let the outer world see the real "me."*

Here, the sufferer's ego is shielding full consciousness by using his body as a preoccupying excuse, keeping him unaware of the deeper psychic conflict because deep within he needs his pain. But he also believes that what he currently understands is all there is to know, as in **egocentric**: *having little or no regard for interests, beliefs, or attitudes other than one's own.* In this instance, his ego is resisting what can ease his suffering because he still requires his pain to keep hidden what he truly wants to say and do (because these feelings and emotions conflict with his culture and societal norms). These norms are usually such things as not caring as much as we feel we should care, or feelings and thoughts of abandoning a relationship or job, being angry at someone we deeply love; not upholding what we have been generally taught to be socially acceptable standards of ethical behavior.

In much rarer instances, they can be thoughts of lust, covetousness, doing serious harm to another, or even harm to self with thoughts of suicide. The intensity of the pain determines the magnitude of danger to the sufferer's personal beliefs, i.e., the standards that he holds himself to—versus—his currently rising darker thoughts and emotions. An individual raised in an austere environment of moral rectitude may be in severe pain after lying about something because they are deeply conflicted in their behavior against the standard they have been raised to adhere to. But another individual who may be openly lying may not be in pain at all if they had been brought up to believe that lying is okay and necessary, on occasion. The difference is in the standard trying to be maintained by the individual, which is constantly monitored by ego.

Ego can be seen influencing, dominating, shielding, and obfuscating daily affairs in other subtle ways, especially in healing. Listed below are some common ways that I've observed.

- "Dr. Sarno talks about knee pain being at the top of the knee, but mine is about a third of an inch below that."

- "I hear people talking about TMS pain at the bottom of the foot all the time, but mine is at the top."

- "I can't find in any of the TMS books, anything about thumb pain."

- "I believe that TMS causes severe back pain, but mine is more like a weak throbbing sensation."

This occurs quite frequently, as each victim of ego attempts to find a way out of all the others' healing scenarios, e.g., "mine is different." Ego does this so that the person can defend the pain, to continue to use the physical body as a shield in order to block the mental. If ego can sabotage healing, then what it desires to hide can stay hidden.

In my first book, I cited four phases of TMS (timings of the onset of pain). I listed the onsets as being, *before, during, returning,* and *after* tension-riddled times. I subsequently received several emails from sufferers saying, "I don't think I fit into any of those times." These poor folks are unconsciously resisting, seeking a way out of healing. Our physical bodies are all the same in most ways. The body is either broken and needs to be repaired, which rarely occurs, or it is reacting to forces that we dare not reveal to anyone, especially to "me."

*My patients often get angry with me when I tell them that they're not as unique as they think they are.*
Marc Sopher, MD, TMS physician, email correspondence

Ego covertly prevents healing by protecting self-image at the cost of unconscious needs. In the process of resisting truth, the body becomes the slave to what the sufferer refuses to be held accountable to.

Ego is also the root word of **egotism**, which is placing oneself at the center—seeing only one view, unable to see other views and opinions. Thus, ego is complex; but in the case of healing, it serves to both shield the sufferer from his personal needs, and to narrow his world down so that he sees only what he wants to see (scotoma).

Bruno Klopfer, PhD, a pioneer in the field of health, psychology, and projective testing (e.g., Rorschach tests), conducted a survey to predict which tumor types, fast-growing or slow-growing, would most likely form, based on individual personality profiles. From the great book, *Getting Well Again*, "The variables that allowed the researchers to predict rapid growth (tumors) were patients' ego defensiveness and loyalty to 'their own version of reality.'" When too much energy is tied up defending the ego and the patient's way of seeing life, the body will not have the necessary vital energy to fight disease. Ego inhibits healing because it steals energy to maintain itself—diverting energy that is needed for healing.

> *If however, a minimum of vital energy is consumed in ego defensiveness, then the cancer has a hard time making headway.*

Bruno Klopfer, PhD[35]

Aldous Huxley, English writer and philosopher, believed that the supreme test of mankind was in overcoming the human disability of egotism. Most of our problems in health as well as in relationships begin with "me"—seeing only our view.

Ego also prevents us from being aware of certain painful emotions such as shame (comparing one's actions to one's standards) by shielding us from our deeper desires. Shame is the love child of perfection and low self-esteem, born into rejection and isolation. In protecting us from shame, ego builds a wall between what we know to be true, and what we pretend to know to be true. The energy spent on deceiving the Self*—through the superego, or persona—creates anger and fatigue. It's within this conflict of pretending to care versus not caring, that pain flourishes.

Psychological conflict is "refereed" by ego, becoming worse by making us think that we are who we're pretending to be.

Advaita spiritual teacher Nisargadatta Maharaj had his life transformed when his guru told him, "You are not what you take yourself to be." Lesson 166 in *A Course in Miracles (ACIM)*[36] states: "This is your chosen self, the one you made as a replacement for reality. This is the self you savagely defend against all reason, and every evidence ... you are not what you pretend to be."

We suffer when we act contrary to what we know to be true; the concept of which psychologist Leon Festinger referred to as **cognitive**

---

*Self: The entire psyche; conscious and unconscious.

**dissonance**. Ego is the referee in this conflict, deciding what we allow others to see of us, what we allow our self to see of ourselves—and in what we accept as being true. Ego then can be seen as truth's gatekeeper. As long as we see ourselves as separate, all knowing, and alone in our feelings, ego is present to govern us. Since we can never rid ourselves entirely of ego, it's more productive in understanding the back pain confusion by focusing on the second leg of EPS: *the wonderful world of placebos.*

## The Power of Mind

In the mid-1990s, I was working with a nationally famous physical therapist for my back pain. He had me aligning my back and body into "proper angles," (remember primal posture) ... and strengthening my core, for back pain relief. At one point, during this realigning and strengthening therapy, I felt and heard a heavy clunking sound ... and my low back and hips seemed to pop into a new position ... my back pain was suddenly gone! I was ecstatic!!! For the first time in my life, that I could remember, my pain was gone. Naturally, I began to praise that therapist to everyone. But my pain returned not long after, and this time, the same therapy wasn't working. In fact, I was getting considerably worse. The truth hadn't risen to light yet; the need to block awareness still existed.

A few years later, after I had recently discovered Dr. Sarno's work and had begun to understand the power of belief, and the placebo-mind, I closed my eyes and envisioned that clunking sound again, recreating the sensation and sound in my mind's eye, and ... my pain instantly left, again. The pain came back worse soon after, but within that moment, I was suddenly aware of the *power of belief* in health. Whenever I would re-envision that clunking sound sensation, and conceptualize my hips and back falling "into primal posture," my pain would stop for a short time, every time. I knew then that all my chiropractic sessions had been placebos. And yet, to this day, people argue over the efficacy of spinal manipulations. They work nicely if you believe in them, but they're not doing anything.

Months later, in the middle of my back-healing campaign, I was jogging down my driveway per the advice of Dr. Sarno to become much more physical. My foot was hurting badly as my brain was trying to shift focus from my back to the bottom of my right foot, in order to keep me down and afraid. At that point I understood TMS, as well as the placebo phenomenon. As I limped down my cement driveway I envisioned, in my mind's eye, that the powder of snow on the driveway was soft cotton, and that my feet were being cushioned as they met the hard pavement. Within a couple seconds my foot pain disappeared and has never returned.

The mind is that powerful—and it cuts both ways. When a physician tells a sufferer that his back is bad, and if the person chooses to accept that archaic notion, that person becomes crippled by his own misguided belief, which is based on the misguided belief of his doctor. Dr. Sarno framed it well in *Healing Back Pain*, "The various health disciplines interested in the back have succeeded in creating an army of the partially disabled in this country with their medieval concepts of structural damage and injury as the basis of back pain[6]."

But there are also those with Howling Dog Syndrome, who see the information on how to heal, but choose to limp around, and rely on support pillows, drugs, physical therapy, and various comfort aids, rather than heal. They accept pain (as decided by their ego), because pain is preferred over facing the unthinkable (revealing more of who they truly are than they want to expose), such as publicly expressing rage, not caring about something or someone, or leaving a job or relationship, among many other possibilities.

We are what we believe, for good or bad. If you believe that your back is a mess, at that point, you truly do have a bad back. Your mindbody will adapt to match your deep belief.

## Procedures Are Placebos

Anyone who has been in back pain, and tried different healing techniques, will already know that some techniques worked for them that didn't work for other sufferers, and vice versa. Some are ecstatic over acupuncture while others never obtain any benefit from it. Some fight to defend spinal manipulations while others get little relief. The same is true for other remedies such as laser surgery, glucosamine and chondroitin, magnets, and epidural injections. Some people love the stuff, while others not so much, which is why the multidisciplinary approach is currently thriving. Placebos are confusing because their outcomes are not related to their apparent causes. Some people are simply pleased by certain techniques so they swear by them as being "the correct way" to heal. It's now clearer than ever, thanks to Dr. Sarno, that some sufferers get relief from certain procedures because they believe it's actually working.* But their temporary relief is based on a complex set of psychological elements.

---

*I have heard the cynics before, "It's because they didn't do the procedure right!" But I, like many, had been to the best and brightest practitioners in their field. The techniques are only as valid as the belief of the sufferer, and have little value beyond conviction.

One such element is the confidence in the **performer** of the ritual which then gets transferred into confidence in the painee, which then yields better results. Another element is **fortunate timing** where the person receiving the treatment is simply having a better day that day, and then wrongly associates the feeling of wellness to the procedure (another spurious correlation). Yet another factor in feeling a sense of false wellness, after a placebo procedure, is the sensory experience surrounding the procedure. People are more heavily influenced, and so tend to feel better if the ritual is technical, powerful, scary, authoritative, and professional-feeling.

Tension-wise, the placebo ritual provides **time away** from the very environment that is triggering the need for the pain in the first place. Many people swear by the spas of The Enchantment in beautiful Sedona, Arizona. They leave their stress-filled jobs and head to the gorgeous desert landscape, and warm sunshine, never quite realizing that the spectacular scenery and time away from their personal warzones is a key ingredient in the potency of the soothing treatments.

We can now look back at the past 100 years or so, and see that most of the medical procedures in the treatment of pain never actually worked, beyond what the individual believed. There are complex psychological factors involved in the process of acceptance and rejection, but a very strong force in the value of any therapeutic technique is **timing**. People suffering, and in desperate need for relief, will latch onto anything they can in their time of despair. Ineffective procedures and worthless advice are more readily accepted by the deeper self when the sufferer has run out of options, and has lost direction. Someone offering hope is a welcoming mechanism in accepting an idea.

*You must remember, my dear lady, the most important rule of any successful illusion: First, the people must want to believe in it.*

Libba Bray[37]

Once again, the proof that procedures like acupuncture and spinal alignment therapy aren't doing anything beyond perceived relief is that once people stop these rituals permanent healing comes. Their minds had been convincing them they were obtaining ongoing relief for several reasons (named above), but the preeminent reason is from a **conditioning process**. If it worked once, it will work again repeatedly, as Pavlov's dogs salivated **every time** upon hearing a bell.

## The Surgery Placebo

The surgery placebo is indeed the most powerful fooling mechanism of all. Surgery is frightening and dangerous, with powerful sensory sounds and smells, and therefore, to the deeper self, is more believable in its effectiveness. We know from Dr. Sarno's successful work that herniated discs don't cause back pain. So when a sufferer feels relief after spinal surgery the odds are excellent that he had a positive response to the performance, as well as, to the performer of the ritual. In thinking he was "corrected," he heals, a little. His belief healed him, along with the "act of surgery," as well as good timing.

Today, small incision laser surgery is popular, and in-vogue. Its current **popularity** provides for a more powerful influence on its effectiveness, for a positive outcome. There are many who respond well to newer techniques, believing they are somehow better than the old ones. Sir William Osler, one of the four founding professors of Johns Hopkins Hospital understood this in the 1800s when he stated, *"One should treat as many patients as possible with a new drug while it still has the power to heal."* Popularity increases the effectiveness of healing techniques.

In the late 1950s, researchers wondered if the technique of tying off damaged arteries (internal mammary ligation[*]) for angina was any better than doing nothing at all for heart patients. So the curious scientists prepared two independent studies in two different US cities to try to understand what was really happening. They had been having success with the ligation surgeries in heart patients but they wanted to know if what they were doing was actually doing anything. So they created two groups. One group got the real ligation surgery and the other got a sham surgery where the participants had an incision in their chest but were sewn up with no surgery. The end results were that the group that had nothing done to them had slightly better improvement (83 percent) compared to the group that had the actual surgery (67 percent)[38]. The "successful" ligation surgeries had been doing nothing all along. The patients' belief that the newfangled procedure was working, with the added scariness of the ritual, made it work.

---

[*]**Internal mammary ligation** surgery, introduced in 1939 by Italian surgeon David Fieschi, was intended to improve bloodflow to the heart for angina pectoris (chest pain).

## Vertebroplasty

Under the same light of consciousness, in February of 2014, I was about to give a lecture on back pain when I saw an article come across the AP on **vertebroplasty**—an amazingly serendipitous discovery on my part. I printed out the article and included it in that night's lecture.

Vertebroplasty is a procedure whereby a special kind of cement is injected into a cracked spinal vertebra. The procedure had been performed in over a million people to relieve pain. The AP article explained how David Kallmes, MD, at the Mayo Clinic had used vertebroplasty for 15 years, and had "found it hugely successful," in healing back pain. But Kallmes noted that there were times that the cement was injected into the wrong vertebra, and the patient healed anyway.

To his credit, Dr. Kallmes set up a clinical trial to see what was actually going on. Half the back pain sufferers received the disc cement and the other half received a fake procedure. The results—predictably— were that the sham surgery participants healed just as quickly as those who got the real vertebral procedure.

A 76-year old female in the trial, whose back was broken with a fractured vertebra was up again and golfing within a week, after receiving the fake procedure. She healed because she believed that she had received the real treatment. She stated that she was certain that she could not be fooled by a sham procedure because she had received the real verte-cement injection the year before after a fall that fractured another vertebra. In the end, she healed just as quickly with no procedure—armed only with the power of her belief.

Regarding the study, Dr. Kallmes stated, "There was no statistically significant difference in degree of pain relief between the patients who underwent vertebroplasty and placebo … and more importantly, there was no statistically significant difference in improvement in function between the patients who underwent vertebroplasty and placebo"[39].

A similar study was being done on vertebroplasty at the same time in Australia, yielding similar results. The million verto-procedures appeared to have not been doing anything beyond misleading sufferers into feeling better. The body heals itself by nature's Grand Design. It rarely needs outside help. However, as we are currently wired, people believe in being medicalized. They feel as though a ritual is necessary for healing to occur; having more faith in science than Nature. But it's even deeper than that. We suffer because we won't accept something we know to be true deep within ourselves, hoping that the "medical acts" will repair our body without having to deal with the unwanted, which is hidden in the body by ego. Medicalizing is an end-run around the real problem; *you can indeed have your fake and treat it, too.*

The same placebo evidence has come forth in knee studies in Finland and from the Baylor College of Medicine, in 2002. The Finnish study, "Arthroscopic Partial Meniscectomy versus Sham Surgery for a Degenerative Meniscal Tear," concluded that, "the outcomes after arthroscopic partial meniscectomy were no better than those after a sham surgical procedure[40]." The lead author of the study, Raine Sihvonen, MD, stated, "By ceasing the procedures (arthroscopic knee surgery to fix a torn cartilage) which have proven ineffective, we would avoid performing 10,000 useless surgeries every year in Finland alone. The corresponding figure for the U.S. is at least 500,000 surgeries."

> *It is we physicians who are responsible for perpetuating false ideas about disease and its cure. The legends are handed along through nurses and fond mothers, but they originate with us, and with every placebo that we give we do our part in perpetuating error, and harmful error at that.*
>
> Richard Cabot, MD[41]

## Is Hope A Placebo?

> *I think 'healing response' is a better term than placebo response.*
>
> Andrew Weil, MD[42]

Bruno Klopfer, PhD, recalls in a 1957 article "Psychological Variables in Human Cancer"[35], the account of a terminally ill patient named Mr. Wright which was communicated to him by Philip West, MD.

Mr. Wright was suffering from lymphosarcoma and had become resistant to all palliative treatments. He had tumors the size of oranges, an enormous spleen and liver, was anemic and on oxygen throughout the day, and had to have fluids drawn from his chest every day. His physicians gave him no hope to live; he was untreatable.

However, Mr. Wright had learned that the clinic he was rapidly dying in was beginning an experimental trial on a new miracle drug called Krebiozen. He wasn't eligible to be in the trial because the study's designers wanted the participants to have a prognosis of six months to live (three months at the minimum), whereas Dr. West felt it was a stretch to expect Mr. Wright to live two more weeks. But when the drug arrived for the trial, Mr. Wright begged Dr. West to let him in, so Dr. West did. Mr. Wright received his first injection on a Friday.

Three days later on Monday, Dr. West returned to the hospital where he expected Mr. Wright to be dead, or at least moribund; then at that point his Krebiozen could be reallocated to another patient.

However, when Dr. West walked in and saw Mr. Wright he was shocked, as Dr. West wrote:

> What a surprise was in store for me! I had left him febrile, gasping for air, completely bedridden. Now, here he was, walking around the ward, chatting happily with the nurses, and spreading his message of good cheer to anyone who would listen. Immediately I hastened to see the others who had received their first injection at the same time. No change, or change for the worse was noted. Only in Mr. Wright was there brilliant improvement. The tumor masses had melted like snowballs on a hot stove, and in only these few days, they were half their original size! ... he (Mr. Wright) had no other treatment other than the single "useless shot."

Ten days after that initial shot of Krebiozen, Mr. Wright was discharged cancer-free and left the hospital to fly his airplane at 12,000 feet. Dr. West described the shot as being "useless" to Klopfer because Krebiozen was later found to be an inert preparation; it had no value. Within two months, reports began emerging publicly that the Krebiozen was useless, with "all of the testing clinics reporting no results." Krebiozen did not work.

Unfortunately, Mr. Wright had been closely monitoring the dismal Krebiozen reports and he quickly began to lose faith in his new miracle drug. Within two months he went from perfect health back to his previous state of terminal disease. At that hapless point, Dr. West decided to take advantage of Mr. Wright's emotional malleability and deliberately lied to him by telling him that there was a better version of Krebiozen arriving that was "super-refined, double-strength." However, since there was no such drug, Dr. West injected Mr. Wright only with fresh water. In Dr. West's words, "Recovery from his second near-terminal state was even more dramatic than the first."

Mr. Wright remained symptom free for two months until he read a report from the American Medical Association stating, "Nationwide tests show Krebiozen to be a worthless drug in treatment of cancer." Within a few days of reading the AMA report, Wright was admitted to the hospital in poor condition and died two days later. *Hope giveth and hope taketh away.*

The importance of this tragic story is in the deeper understanding of why so many people feel that their back surgery, or any other spinal technique worked for them, when it most likely has done nothing. Their belief that it would work, and did work, through their confidence in their surgeon had transformed their physiology by providing hope. The mind is limitless in its capacity to transform expectations. The proof that most back pain sufferers don't need surgery is that virtually all of those who come to understand TMS and why they have their pain, heal.

As Dr. Sarno stated, most medical studies are inaccurate if they don't consider emotions, and I would also add sufferers' personal beliefs to his statement because the only thing that matters in healing is what the sufferer wants and needs.

Emotions are the effects of needs and wants. When back pain sufferers attempt various treatments like trigger point therapy, gua sha, Rolfing, Feldenkrais, Cox Flexion Distraction, and the Alexander, Thompson, Gonstead, and Bowen techniques, among innumerable others, they are looking for that thing that pleases them. If they eventually find what they want, their pain may ease some. The techniques themselves are bolstered by confidence in the performer. However the healing techniques also provide sensory stimuli to compete with the pain for awareness. And so techniques like gua sha shift the sufferer's mind's eye toward the "scratchings," which divert the senses away from the pain. Spinal manipulation, core strengthening, spinal aligning, and stretching techniques make the sufferer feel better sometimes, but quite often only temporarily.

Our beliefs define who we are. The expectation of a given treatment gets screened through our belief-set which wills the body into healing, worsening, or no change. Mr. Wright probably strongly believed in medications, but he may also have been so desperate at that point that he was willing to latch onto anything that conveyed hope. Thus, his tragic story provides some great teaching moments on placebos, healing, and belief. The placebo's effectiveness:

- Is increased if it reduces worry to the point of relaxation so that real healing can take place;
- Depends on ritual;
- Is correlated with desperation, i.e., the "Wright timing";
- Can bring about a permanent cure if the cause of the dis-order is dealt with simultaneously;
- Is greater in certain personalities who "buy in" more readily;
- Increases with trust in the performer of the ritual;
- Depends almost entirely on positive programming (expectations of success).

Bernie S. Siegel, MD, writes in his extraordinary book *Love, Medicine, and Miracles*, that "Negative programming is one reason why a fourth of all chemotherapy patients start throwing up before they get to their next treatment. In England a group of men were given saline and told it was chemotherapy, 30 percent had their hair fall out"[43]. Of course negative programming can be counteracted with positive programming, which is exactly what a placebo is; a positive action. The placebo provides a sense of control over the pain or disease, whereas the sufferer previously felt no control. But it has little effect if the patient doesn't trust in the practitioner or the process. The same is true for psychotherapy.

There are many well-documented placebo stories of healing through positive programming, as well as tragic nocebo events triggered by negative programming. There are also incalculable odd and interesting chronicled stories of health and healing belief, such as:

- People taking the wrong pill to stop their nausea and the nausea disappearing even though the pill that was taken was known to cause nausea.

- The late Norman Cousins, PhD, spoke of a conversation he overheard between two oncologists comparing their protocols for administering chemotherapy. The first oncologist told his patients he was giving them EPOH from the first letters of the chemo-drug combination, etoposide, Platinol, Oncovin, and hydroxyurea, and had a 22% success rate in healing. The second oncologist, who was using the same combination of drugs, but emphasized his protocol as HOPE, had a 74% success rate[44].

- As reported in the Scottish Daily Record, a Scottish dancer named Antonia DiCarlo claimed she was healed from two years of agonizing back pain by the technique of gua sha. The headline of the article reads, "Dancer who suffered years of agonising back pain cured using the lid from a honey jar." Antonia no doubt felt relief from the ritual, but she might not know how powerful her beliefs were in her healing. A honey jar lid certainly cannot heal a real structural spinal problem, and so her relief points directly to her pain being psychological in nature (TMS), and to the placebo phenomenon. If there were any physical benefits from the ritual it would further prove Dr. Sarno correct that TMS pain stems from a reduction in oxygen to the nerves, muscles, and tendons. Gua sha practitioners assert that the procedure stimulates blood flow for healing (microcirculation), and the "bruising" clearly creates a competing stimulus to the obsession on the pain (a new diversion)[45].

Gua sha appears to be further proof that it is not the spine itself that is causing these painful conditions but rather the thought and belief processes.

Odd scenarios in health seem endless; such as those individuals with split personalities as reported in the Science section of the New York Times in May of 1985. A woman with a split personality while in one of her personalities was diabetic, but "showed no symptoms of the disorder" in her other personality. A man with a split personality was allergic to fruit juices in one personality but not in another[46]. The power of the mind in health and healing is awe-inspiring.

However, the blade that opens the gap of understanding has two edges in a world of dualistic turmoil ... **and the yin chases the yang as this becomes that**. As long as physicians and alternative healers keep telling back pain sufferers that they have bad spines, and that they need to do this or to do that to heal, the suffering will continue through the nocebo effect. In almost all cases, the spine does not need anything done to it to heal from back pain. Nothing. I have heard many times from back pain sufferers, "I feel like I need to DO something." But they don't. The lesson of this book is one of revelation, not of "what to do." Trying to heal is the number one mistake made in healing from back pain.

She wants to be pleased when she is in fear for her health. And so she will clasp onto anything that she feels may work. If her belief is deep enough then any process might work. However, once the procedure pleases her she mistakenly feels she truly had a spinal problem, but the root cause remains lurking, waiting to rise again when needed. Placebo healing can be superficial since it doesn't always reach far enough into the mindbody to exact permanent change. Permanent healing occurs when the truth is accepted and the transforming life work is done.

If I had a magic wand and could wave it over "Joe Common pain sufferer" to take away his pain, his pain would return soon after if his thinking patterns and beliefs don't change. As long as he reacts to his daily life and his relationships in the same way, he is not fully healed, even though his pain is gone. Therefore, all the placebo healing techniques imagined to date are more often temporary (the Symptom Imperative being one measure of a placebo's success). The healing techniques simply temporarily divert awareness, shifting consciousness, until the brain once again needs help to keep the individual distracted.

There is massive confusion over how to heal because the entire back pain industry is made up of various placebo approaches and well-intended professionals, some of which can be highly convincing. But the only way to heal permanently has been proven to work on the psychological aspects of the need for the pain. And of course nearly everyone in the pain industry is against that notion because it requires no body solutions.

The highest permanent back pain healing rate is through TMS healing, which by default advances the greatest hope. Even though hope pleases, it is not a placebo in itself. Hope is the light within that kindles the spark of life. The mechanisms that hope utilizes may be placebos, if they give us what we want, at the correct time. The phrase "just a placebo effect" has been used often in a denigrating fashion. But Mr. Wright certainly didn't care how his healing occurred; he was happy to be alive. And so now, Dr. Weil is correct, "healing response" is the better perspective on the healing rituals; armed with the knowledge that the cause of pain and disease remains, post-ritual, if not attended to, or even worse not recognized.

## The Modern Era of Medicine and its Sham Wows

With each **positive placebo result**, and **subsequent symptom shift**, the sufferer is deceived into believing that there was initially a structural problem, and that modern medical techniques hold the answers to all healing … and the confusion continues. It's within these false healings that epidemics develop.

When I hear the admonitions: "I have a bad back," or, "I have a disc problem," or even worse, "My doctor told me …." it always makes me cringe. For 30 years I believed those same false notions. But I was also once a victim of the great pain deception.

I've taught people how to recover from severe pain in many countries, thanks to the good doctor, Dr. Sarno. Once they heal, they invariably ask the same question, "Why doesn't anyone know about TMS?" They try to tell their friends and family, and they get laughed at. They're roundly and soundly rejected because many find the TMS solution to suffering insulting. I've been chastised too many times with the statement, "You're insulting my intelligence with this crap!" But intelligence cannot be insulted. It is ignorance that gets insulted. Intelligence is open and ready for change—willing to listen to anything that will add to the greater good of the Self. That's why it's intelligent: it expands through learning. Ignorance is the thing that won't let go, the thing that gets stung.

**Intelligence:** *the faculty of understanding, a capacity for learning, reasoning, understanding, an aptitude in grasping truths, relationships, facts, meanings.*

Marc Sopher, MD, co-author of *The Divided Mind—The Epidemic of Mindbody Disorders*, described a patient who stormed out of his office when told that his low back pain was most likely emotionally induced. The patient insisted that his pain was "real pain."* The patient came back two days later and apologized, telling Dr. Sopher that, because Dr. Sopher had stuck with him and his family through tough times over the years, he was willing to listen to what he had to say. The man read

---

*The act of storming out is a sign of deep rage, as well as a defensive technique to keep the real cause hidden. Walk toward your problems, not away.

Dr. Sarno's *Healing Back Pain*, along with some other TMS information, and his "pain simply vanished."

## Shifting Truth

I received an email from a lady telling me that spinal surgery worked great for her, and that TMS healing is just selling a quack remedy to desperate people. I responded by asking her, "If your surgery worked great, then why are you still reading and researching information on how to heal back pain?" She responded back by saying that she still has pain, but that, "My doctor didn't do the surgery right"—followed by—"Surgery is still the answer!"

These people are drawn into some type of sick game of scapegoating and self-sabotage that ego lures them into—shifting blame through displacement. **Displacement** is an unconscious psychological defense mechanism used where the person unconsciously redirects her unwanted emotions and desires toward something else, such as another person, jogging, phobias, cleaning, working, joking, and blaming. The German word for displacement, verschiebung, means "to shift." Shifting blame allows them to assuage their own guilt by bypassing their ego, making them feel better about themselves. In this case, the spine is getting the blame for the problems in people's lives, because ego won't admit that anything is wrong.

Ego is at the center of scapegoating, and at the very heart of most of our problems, especially our health problems, as shown with EPS:

**Ego:** Denies the truth, hides the shame, disguises the conflicts, projects the weaknesses, and rejects the solutions

**Placebo:** Temporarily pleases, altering physiology

**Symptom shifting:** Keeps people confused because they feel the last problem was solved, but in reality it was simply pushed somewhere else

## Okay, Let's Say This Crap Is True—Now What??

If you're reading this, then you either have back pain or you're trying to help someone you love who is in pain. If you're having trouble healing, then you've probably been focusing on the wrong things—like I did, for three decades. If you've injured your back it will heal in a few days, weeks, or months. Your pain will not continue in perpetuity. It will end after the emotional process is **recognized**, accepted and dealt with, and the **conditioning** process is **interrupted**.

If you decide not to believe in something that can take your pain away, then you should try to understand why you're protecting your pain. The answers should be more obvious by now, but people always have questions. These are the best questions I've heard so far.

## Q and A:

- **I bent over and heard a loud "pop." Are you telling me that my back is okay?** Yes, the pop meant nothing, unless you tore the structure of your spine apart. The popping sound may reveal some tension and is a trigger for your brain to initiate pain. The brain was ready at that time for a diversion. If you had truly injured your back it would have healed in a short time. If it was a real injury, the pain would have ended fairly soon.

- **I saw my x-rays with osteoarthritis. Are you trying to tell me that arthritis isn't causing my pain?** Yes. Osteoarthritis doesn't cause pain. If it did, your pain would be there all the time, non-stop.

- **Why did I feel better right after surgery, and then got worse?** The rituals and fear surrounding the surgery replaced the obsession on the spine. The surgery becomes a replacement obsession, for a short time, as it takes the intense focus off the pain and diverts it toward the worry over the surgery. Once the fear-focus on the surgery fades, the pain returns because the surgery didn't do anything. If the pain does not return, the brain has fully accepted that the procedure worked ... and ... the necessity for the diversion has ended.

- **If the causes of pain are unknown to me, how can I acknowledge them?** It's not necessary to find "the source," or a specific cause of the pain. It would help, but it's not mandatory, and is rarely possible. It's more important to become aware of the thoughts and emotions that are generating the rage. In other words, your childhood is in the past, your personality has formed. You now react and respond to daily events through the prism you have formed over time, and learned to live by. That prism, of personality and memory experience, generates great rage due to a complex web of behavioral characteristics based on shame and unmet personal needs. Becoming aware of all of this is *the process of healing*.

  Events can't be undone, but emotional attachment to them can be released, as well as the current responses to events. Letting go, forgiving freely, and understanding the mindbody process free the energy held in the form of fear, rage, and resentment. Rage can sometimes be expressed away, but that's rarely needed in healing. Rage can dissipate through self-awareness, which is the more common way of healing.

- **If herniations don't cause back pain, then why did my surgery work?** My first response to this question is always, "If it worked, then why are you still researching and reading about back pain?" If it did work, though, it would be for one of two reasons: 1) your deeper brain believed it worked; or more rarely, 2) you didn't have TMS. If you had pinched a nerve you would have been paralyzed quickly. At which point your pain would have ended once the nerve died. Dead nerves cannot transmit pain signals.

- **How do I tell someone about TMS without getting my head ripped off?** The best way is to tell them about you; relay your story, and don't preach to them about their pain. If you preach, their first reaction is normally to become ego-defensive and to take a stronger stance against truth. It's a waste of time trying to convert people; it doesn't work. For some reason, explaining the Symptom Imperative seems to be less offensive to sufferers, most likely because all the psychosomatic jargon is bypassed. But also perhaps because they can observe its effects directly in its movements. A friend also noticed that sufferers are more likely to listen to the explanation of what he calls the "ping pong effect" of the symptoms, rather than to a direct affront to their ego, drawing their psyche into question. Truth cannot be foisted upon people, only realized from within. When they're **ready** to accept it, they will. Dr. Sarno advised me, "Steve, spend your time and energy on helping those who are willing to listen; there's enough of them out there." He was right, again.

- **Is it possible that my spine's structure could cause my back pain?** Yes. Anything is possible. I saw a woman on Discovery Channel that was her own twin. She had two sets of DNA in her body, making her, her own sister. Odd things happen in nature, and the spine can have some bizarre abnormalities that may need correction. It's not likely, but it's certainly possible. If you haven't lost control of your bowel and bladder, or are currently not paralyzed, then your spine is probably okay. However, be aware, my left leg was partially paralyzed, and I lost my deep tendon reflexes. I lost feeling, movement, and sensation, with drop foot—and yet I had TMS. Neurosurgeons, general practitioners, and orthopedic surgeons consistently told me that I had a pinched nerve, and bad spine. They were all wrong.

- **Can you have both TMS and pain from a spinal defect?** No. You either have a structural problem, or you have TMS. If there's a structural problem causing pain, then that's not TMS. However, with any illness or physical pain, there also exists a psychological component. If you injure yourself your anxiety and anger will naturally rise, aggravating the injury. But emotions aren't the cause of that pain, they're only adding to its intensity. If you have TMS, it only appears that you have a structural problem, but you don't. Very few people have real spinal problems, but most think they do.

- **Can I take medication and heal?** Yes, and no. How's that for clarity? This one is tricky because an artificial element is being introduced. Drugs may prevent full healing by inhibiting the cognitive changes necessary to uproot old beliefs, and replacing old beliefs with more accurate beliefs is how to heal. There have also been people who healed as soon as they stopped taking their meds. Their medications had been triggering their pain in an **association response**, like Pavlov's pups and the ringing bells. In this case, the meds were the bell, and the pain was the salivating. The brain senses the chemical and thinks it should create pain. Stopping the medication in these cases stopped the chemically triggered pain response by breaking the association.

   It's also important to understand that your body's equilibrium can become so far out of balance that you may need medication to regain a sense of control. Don't feel guilty for having to take them, but also be aware of any unconscious need for them. If you refuse to ever get off your medication, try to understand why you need to hide your emotional pain, which will be the same reason you need your physical symptoms. But there are many types of medications for different purposes. Only your doctor knows why she or he has placed you on them, so never just stop medicating, suddenly. Be careful.

   ✓ This is also a good time to make the lawyers happy. This book is not a substitute for a medical exam. I'm not a doctor, nor am I qualified to hand out medical advice. Me don't know nothen. I'm only reporting on all that I've seen, in order to help someone— anyone—who is willing to listen. When I give out TMS advice I assume the sufferer has been medically cleared for life-threatening disorders. TMS is harmless, cancer may not be.

- **Is it possible that my spinal discs are slipping in and out, causing my back pain?** No, that is structurally impossible. The notion that discs slip, however, has allowed many folks to slip in and out of the bank to cash big checks. More and more "spinal manipulators" are now agreeing that it's impossible to slip a disc. As a preemptive measure, some are now replacing the term "disc slipping" with the term "joint slipping." But there's no such thing as joint slipping either. It's simply repackaging of an old myth.

- **Is it possible to hurt my back lifting something that was too heavy to lift?** No, as Dr. Sarno said, "If it was too heavy to lift you couldn't have lifted it." You can of course hurt your back lifting something that was not too heavy to lift, but your back will heal. Lifting and bending are proven to be triggers of pain, and are normally not damaging to the spine.

- **Is it possible to heal even if you've had spinal surgery, or multiple surgeries?** Yes, it doesn't matter how many surgeries you've had, you can still heal. Spinal surgery doesn't damage the spine (unless the surgeon makes a serious mistake). Healing is always possible if you consciously desire to do so—and then from that point, your stubborn unconscious begins the necessary change. It must also be stated that scarring from spinal surgery does not cause trouble in healing (unless the person believes it does).

- **Please, if there was just ONE thing? One simple thing that you could tell me that would help me right now! I'm suffering terribly. Before I start to read all the TMS material, what would the ONE thing be to help me?** Sadly, I get this question too often from people in great suffering. The answer is *conscious breathing*. The first step in gaining control over pain is conscious breathing. Belly breathing. Soothe yourself.

- **Please, if there was just ONE book? One book that could help me. I'm so confused with all this health stuff. Which book would you recommend?** Although I healed primarily with *Healing Back Pain*, and I believe that it's all that anyone needs in order to heal, my personal belief is that *The Will to Live* is the best health book yet written. Although to anyone currently suffering, it's probably too much of the big picture, too soon, in order to help. The psyche is only able to absorb great truths in small doses. For instant relief, *Healing Back Pain* is "the book," and has been proven highly effective when coupled with *The Great Pain Deception*. Together they appear to have formed a dynamic duo. For the end game in healing, *The Will to Live* was simply and elegantly written; encapsulating the many reasons for pain and illness. Here are a few summations from its Chapter 10. Keep in mind that this book was written in 1951[47]. Its author, Arnold Hutschnecker, MD, graduated in 1925, two years after Dr. Sarno was born. The truth has been around since the beginning, but gets tarnished in self-interest. As you read these summation statements substitute the word "illness" with "back pain."

  ✓ Illness may come as a needed respite from problems we feel unable to solve, perhaps unable to face.

  ✓ Illness may be an unconscious device to change a situation by influencing another's attitude or behavior toward us.

✓ Illness may be a way to give vent to hostility that we cannot accept within ourselves and so must suppress.

✓ Illness may be acute, a way of getting out of a temporarily difficult situation, or it may become chronic, if the situation continues to be unresolved.

- **Do I have to quit my job or get a divorce to heal?** No, not normally, but it depends on how debilitated you are. Pain is a fairly normal experience—it's universal, part of the human condition. If you're in a wheelchair, or bedridden, you may want to consider severing any ties that bind you to your rage. Your current relationship, or career, may not be the path that your deeper self wants to be traveling on. However, it's important to know that "leaving" does not always solve the problem; it only releases the trigger. How you react to life remains the same, nothing has changed. By leaving, you haven't healed; you've only temporarily released the pain.

## The Real Causes of Back Pain

The relationship arguments, rejections, deaths of loved ones, financial worries, lack of pleasure, mid-life crisis, anxiety over aging and health, life disappointments, and loneliness are the main causes of back pain. These psychological events are perceived rejections, shames, isolations, and disconnects—separations—that provoke enormous rage within. The rage is the social reaction to the fear of being alone (isolated/rejected). However, the anger from these events is never felt (experienced) by the sufferer because ego casts it outside of awareness and into the spine, or other body areas. It's that direct, and excruciatingly painful.

I've witnessed people who were bedridden and others in wheelchairs that stayed in their jobs, and with their spouses, who healed with this knowledge. They became aware of, and accepted, that they themselves were creating their pain, based on how they were "not reacting" to their lives. The only change they needed was within, not from a divorce, or new career. But for other sufferers, leaving helped them begin to heal.

To heal, you need to know there are powerful emotions beneath your awareness that exist, and then begin to connect the pain to those emotions by seeing the pain as an emotion, and not as a spine problem. These emotions are a side of you that your ego refuses to accept. I've had people tell me that they were thrilled with their new therapist, because she or he told them "everything they wanted to hear!" But that's not always a good sign. It is those things we don't want to hear that are causing the suffering. The relationship with the therapist is the more important aspect, one of compassion, and trust. Sometimes the therapist has to relay aspects of the sufferer's life he isn't aware of, and doesn't want to hear, but in a way that the ego won't get threatened. Helping is an art-form.

Healing from back pain encompasses seeing a side of yourself that you don't want to admit to. This is a truth that many people steadfastly refute, but remains steadfastly true.

*The truth will set you free, but first it will piss you off.*
Gloria Steinem

# 7

# Emotions

## Shame: The Most Painful Emotion

Guilt helps us to remain good people. Shame is a social rejection that isolates us. These are normal reactions at various stages of life. The brain creates back pain to protect us from sensing our degrees of guilt and shame. When these painful emotions become perilously close to being recognized, the brain increases the pain to intolerable states in order to prevent their awareness. The more aware that sufferers become of this process, the better they tend to heal. The resistance to the notion of psychosomatic* pain is due to the epic fight by ego to protect self-image from embarrassment, and the resistance to accepting any truth emanates from this same ego involvement.

People are ashamed of their fear and anger. They're ashamed of wanting to leave their family, or quit a job, or that they really don't care about someone. They're ashamed of how they look, what they need, or what they have, or don't have. Within that shame they have deep guilt, as good people, because they know they shouldn't feel that way. The sufferer who doesn't understand this is usually the one who has the most problem healing. We all feel guilt and shame, followed by disappointment. The end result of these conflicts within the mind is toxic rage, driven by fear, followed by more guilt, and more shame. This is one aspect of the shadow-self.

Our shadow is the black side of our personality. We simply don't want to believe we have one. Everything that the shadow is, the person has no wish to be, and so many deny that it even exists in them. But as Dr. Jung learned and stated, "Everyone carries a shadow, and the less it is embodied in the individual's conscious life, the blacker and denser it is[48]." When we won't admit to these shadow thoughts, or at least that they exist, our shadow becomes even more powerful over us, and the pain increases accordingly. Back pain protects us from becoming aware of the rage that results from panic, guilt, and shame. But, it's all hidden by ego, thus the pain.

**Shame:** *a feeling of guilt, regret, or sadness that you have because you feel you have done something wrong.*

---

*"Psychosomatic" is the earlier term for mindbody. Both terms are used interchangeably, but mindbody is less offensive.

## Helen

In his book, *The Mindbody Prescription*, Dr. Sarno tells the story of Helen who was bedridden, "paralyzed with pain," as her shadow began to possess her. At 47, she had remembered being molested by her father, and joined an incest support group to try to heal her wounds. As she entered the support group her symptoms began to worsen. She couldn't understand why she was getting worse but her husband insightfully pointed out to her, "You're talking about forty years of repressed anger." His words suddenly triggered an emotional catharsis as she cried harder than she had ever cried in her life, as she described, "out-of-control tears." She began blurting out words such as "let me die, I feel sick, I'm so afraid, please take care of me." Her shadow then began to fade in the light of truth. She described her pain leaving her like a pipeline from her lower back through her eyes, pouring out of her. Her pain initially began to increase—as it often does—to prevent certain emotions from entering consciousness. In the end, the truth set her free as her pain had no more purpose, since it had only existed to aid in the denial of her shame, and the fury behind the darker thoughts that brought on that shame.

Helen's example is a most dramatic and direct example of how back pain serves to protect us. Instances of this magnitude are rare, but it illustrates the TMS process elegantly. Most back pain sufferers weren't molested, although some in severe pain have told me they wondered if they had been, and had blocked it from their memory. They then began searching for things that didn't exist. Most of the guilt and shame driving the need for pain usually surround wanting to quit something or leave something, cheat on someone, harm someone, not care about someone, and from not feeling worthy (self-hate), or feeling as a failure. Shame is a separation, an emotional death.

Spouses commonly experience unconscious separation rage in the form of severe back pain if their spouse dies, or even during divorce. Once they recognize that the child primitive in them was angry at their spouse for leaving them alone, they tend to heal. The shame and loneliness of being angry at someone for leaving becomes unbearable. There is an infinite set of other possibilities, and combinations surrounding pain from abandonment rage, such as, the shame and fear of having an illness, rejections from criticisms, and of not feeling good enough. Some of the back pains from guilt and shame stem from suicidal thoughts, and darker images. All fear comes from the isolation of darkness. All rage* stems from fear, and to the strong attachment to "I."

---

*Some chemicals can cause rage. Rage here refers to a mindbody response to separation.

We know from experience that these darker thoughts are indeed present in the sufferers, due to the great successes in treatment. The psychological aspects behind the creation of pain can get quite complex, but the "cure" doesn't have to be. Healing from pain doesn't have to be a long drawn-out process. It can occur fairly quickly. However, slower healing appears to be psychologically safer, and often leads to a more permanent healing. Slow healing is okay, and normal, and not necessarily a sign of a problem. But in life there are always fine lines. Slow healing may also mean the sufferer is putting off the needed work: delaying healing, protecting the pain. Balance is king.

## The Dilemma of the Current System

What's going on in the sufferer's life is almost never considered in the evaluation of pain. By that, I mean, there are almost no medical doctors who look at the sufferer's life events, personality, family history, and thinking process—before prescribing a worthless body solution.* Medical systems around the world simply aren't set up to heal; they're designed to treat broken bodies. It should also be noted that most medical doctors wouldn't know what to do with the information even if it was obtained. They're generally not psychologists, or psychiatrists. They're not trained to understand the mindbody. On the other side, psychologists and therapists aren't trained in medicine, so they're not in the business of diagnosing. Thus, there's a gap problem in healthcare systems between body and mind. Dr. Sarno filled that gap by developing a team to work together on the pain dilemma—and his team won.

The perfunctory routine is to take imaging, point to something in the body as the problem, inject, medicate, stretch, strengthen, or cut. This is a model that has been proven to fail, if only by the fact that back pain is the #1 cause of job disability. Treating back pain and healing back pain are mutually exclusive goals—if you have TMS, you cannot do both: treat your back AND heal. **You have to choose one or the other: treat it or heal it.** All the therapeutic techniques are paradoxically assisting your brain with its ploy to bury the unwanted. To heal, you have to focus only on your emotions ... which emanate from your thinking process. This new awareness diffuses the pain in an elegant manner, and has been labeled by Dr. Sarno as "thinking psychologically."

---

*Many are now complaining that their doctors don't even look at them during the office visit. The physician walks in and heads over to the charts, scribbles a new script, and walks out.

# 8

# Imitating and Reflecting Suffering

## Simulacrum and Hyperreality

Ulcers were once more prevalent than in today's society. As the **collective consciousness** of society became aware that ulcers were due to stress, and came to collectively accept that they emanated mainly from an emotional process (and not from defective stomachs) the ulcer as a health distraction necessarily had to shift. Society then needed a new "collectively agreed upon place of concern" (diversion) in which to hide its problems. People continually need a physical outlet in which to hide undesirable and overwhelming thoughts and emotions. The coping mechanism utilized will sometimes be the one that the person next to them has—the one that's okay to have without shame, at that time in society. The diversions more often come from those we observe around us: the new **observance coping mechanism**.

> **Simulacrum:** *a material image, likeness, similarity, representation or imitation, without the substance or proper qualities of the original.*

> **Hyperreality:** *the inability of consciousness to distinguish reality from a copy or simulation of reality.*

**This doesn't mean that you can't hurt your back**! Au contraire mon ami. The pain is real and you can indeed hurt yourself, sometimes badly. **Observance coping mechanism** here means: *he is aware of a problem, so he has certain expectations of it.*

Regarding back pain:

- He expects: to have back pain after a popping sound.
- He expects: his healing may take longer.
- He expects: medical attention may be required.
- He expects: there to be an ongoing problem there.

Within his **expectations** he paves a new road for his future suffering, not his pain. His pain is real—the extent of his suffering is partially determined by his observations. What he observes, he expects, and is therefore acceptable for him to use when he needs a socially acceptable place to bury what he feels he needs to hide from others—to avoid rejection.

The common migraine serves the same "distractionary" purpose as the ulcer, and back pain. However, now people collectively understand that most migraines are the result of tension. They have properly linked the onset of migraines to daily events in their lives (the Tiger Woods conundrum). Generally speaking, society understands that migraines are not a body problem, but rather stress related. There can be more serious reasons for migraines, of course; but generally speaking, people have come to the awareness that migraines are harmless effects of emotions. Now, at that **point of awareness**, the migraine lost most of its authority as an anger diversion. A diversion is only a diversion as long as the person isn't aware that it's a diversion.

"Migraines dropped a foot" is the earlier catch phrase for this concept. This means the migraine, as an emotional diversion dropped about a foot's distance down the body from the head to the stomach. The brain then began to use stomach ulcers as a new focal point of worry, the new diversion post-migraines. The "worry" is in the notion that something is wrong with the body, and that it needs to be repaired. This is an important point. By using the words **worry**, and **focus**, and **obsession**, and **diversion**, I mean that people believe they need a doctor to repair these problems because they feel that their body has failed, or is somehow breaking down.* However, as we pull back further for a better look, these things that we once felt needed repairing, we now see were only masquerading as broken body parts, as diversions. And the very act of forcing them into the "needs repaired" category perpetuated the original deception. The problems then became epidemic because the ego-brain created her problems, hoping that she would focus on fixing her body, which is, with forethought, her brain's intent.

Continuing down the body, so to speak, as society grew to understand that these problems were effects of reactions to life, and that the body was okay, the problems continued to shift. Our very act of observing them had altered the way we were responding to them.

---

*It can also allow the sufferer to connect with the physician when they are overwhelmed, and nobody at home is there for them to lean on. The physician acts as a surrogate for their deep need to feel safe, heard, and connected.

# Foot Drop

Dr. Sarno connected the dots even further by mentioning how back pain had replaced ulcers, when he pointed to the 1981 New York Times Magazine column, "Where Have All the Ulcers Gone?" As ulcers became less of a concern regarding structural defects in the stomach—a new place of concern needed to arise, and that place was in the **postural muscles**, mainly low back pain. Hence, the emotional diversion dropped yet another foot from the stomach to the low back.

Traveling farther down the body, TMS physician Marc Sopher stated in his book, *To Be or Not to Be ... Pain-Free*, that he believed foot pain was the new popular diversionary pain disorder (TMS). Twenty-five years earlier, in the early years of his medical practice, no one came into his office complaining of foot pain. Two-and-a-half decades later, many folks were limping in and complaining of painful feet. We have the best footwear ever designed in history, to comfort and support our feet. It doesn't make sense that the structure of the human foot would have suddenly collapsed, and is now causing an explosion of foot pain. The answer, as Dr. Sopher knows well, is that people are observing other people in foot pain, and then reflecting and magnifying the problem through the news, workplace, media, friends, and family— through social observation.

Of course, somewhere between the migraine and foot problems, are the diversions of shoulder, knee, hand, and ankle pain—most of which are TMS. It's difficult to find a more unnecessary business than routine rotator cuff surgery on healthy shoulders that have only normal wear and tear, and surgery on healthy knees that have natural wearing and tearing. However, back surgery on innocuous disc problems currently tops the list of unnecessary procedures.

As we become more aware of the brain's survival strategy, not only in where it creates the new distractions, but in its NEED to create a new distraction, the problem will necessarily shift from head to toe, and back again. In Dr. Sopher's observations, society has discovered a new hiding place, lower than the low back: the feet! It could be said then, that the migraine has dropped once again—but this time, "two more feet."

When people "become aware" that a symptom is not a body problem, but rather the survival brain diverting awareness to the body—the symptoms must shift to keep them guessing as to which problem is a real structural problem to worry about, and which is a mindbody effect pretending to be a structural problem. Observation and awareness affect the outcome by uncovering the charade. The uncovering of what is actually occurring either initiates healing, or it forces yet another symptom shift.

## Memes and Social Replication

> *Meme theory suggests that items of gossip are like living things that seek to reproduce using humans as their host.*
>
> Amy Farrah Fowler, PhD, "Big Bang Theory"

Symptoms are potentially contagious through **memetic infection**. All the meme needs is a **host**—and then, an unsuspecting victim whose emotions are threatening to overwhelm them, someone who currently needs to be infected.

Our needs often overwhelm us in a silent manner, and sometimes the only way to express the isolation is through the physical body. That physical expression can take an infinite variety of forms. And oftentimes, the fear of isolation and rejection is assuaged through unconsciously **mimicking** what those around us are suffering from, in the instinctual need to feel connected. When we feel powerless over our current situation, and have no one to express our anger to, our instincts seek ways to stay connected. The deeper-self understands that the resolution of conflict, and ultimately healing, comes through **connection**.

## The Rotating Hall of Mirrors

Connection to others is our **most basic instinct**, and by default our deepest need. Connection is the opposing state of rejection. We fill this need to be connected through our senses. If we don't sense that we are connected, safe, loved, or needed, the body begins to tear itself apart, in many imaginable ways. The deeper the sense of detachment the greater the price the body pays. Pioneering psychiatrist Clancy D. McKenzie, author of, *Babies Need Mothers*, has stated that the internal rage is directly proportional to how helpless we are at the time we feel separate, or feel abandoned. Sometimes people use violent outbreaks of murder to express their rage at the fear of detachment. Sometimes they try to be perfect, or nice, to avoid any possible disconnect. There are never-ending ways to try to connect, and they all come through being heard (recognized). If the unconscious goal in connecting is to fit in, to comply—the connection method may be right in front of us. And it's not always a conscious decision; rather, it can be accomplished through memetic contagion.

Whether it's ulcers or back pain, what we observe in others will be the new *digression-du-jour* because others give us permission for it.

"Others" are the current meme hosts, the ones we're observing and imitating, as reflected in Richard Rohr's notion of a *rotating hall of mirrors*. We aren't fully aware that our senses are constantly observing and parroting life around us—"sub"-consciously absorbing, imitating, and reflecting our surroundings. We continually reflect our own lives back to ourselves, all the truths and the errors; but we also catch and mix in others' behaviors—their truths and their errors. The greatest illusion of all time is that we are separate beings.

**Observational learning:** *imitating others' behaviors through observing them.*

## What's Trending

From my own research, the newest emergent diversionary epidemic looks to be hand pain. I've received hundreds of emails from people with hand and wrist pain: from musicians, secretaries, doctors, construction workers, and teenagers. The fastest-growing within this group appears to be the texting-video-gamers—mostly males in the 20 to 45 age group. People use high-tech devices quite often as a means of alleviating and diverting anxiety. They're unaware that the stress and tension they're trying to mitigate is being diverted to their hands and wrists because "the brain will NOT be denied!" The stressors they're attempting to divert by obsessing on technical devices are being diverted to their hands and wrists, in the form of tension.

Later, when their tension reaches an overflow point and their hands and wrists become too painful to use, their doctors may diagnose them as having carpal tunnel (CT), or repetitive strain injury (RSI), or complex regional pain syndrome (CRPS)—the very terms the doctors themselves have created in order to define the pain, and to capitalize on it. In the defining of it, they legitimize it, and in its legitimizing they magnify it; and in the magnifying of it, it spreads through social imitation.

Anxiety that isn't dealt with properly will rear its shaky hand somewhere, and that somewhere is either a place that is "unconsciously suggested" to be vulnerable through observation—OR— in the body part that's most involved in the conscious repetitive process. Skeptics will say, "Well ... they're over-using that body part. Of course it's going to wear out and hurt!"* The simplest response to that statement is still, "no." The proof, once again, that they are wrong is in the fact that these people heal once they realize they're holding tension

---

*Did you ever notice how skeptics and naysayers always use exclamation points!!

in their hands and wrists, and do the mental work to overcome the cause. We are simply not that weak as human beings or we would have never survived this long.

There is an obvious hand and wrist pain problem, that a couple decades ago was being blamed on the rise of computer use. But humans worked much harder, and longer, with their hands in the past. Finally, in 2006, a Harvard University study debunked the myth of computer use as the cause of damage to the hands and wrists.

> *Report Summary: The popular belief that excessive computer use causes painful carpal tunnel syndrome has been contradicted by experts at Harvard Medical School. According to them, even as much as seven hours a day of tapping on a computer keyboard won't increase your risk of this disabling disorder.*
>
> Harvard University[49]

Computers are fairly easy on the hands and in no way have harmed the hands and wrists. The problem is in the rise in tension that gets targeted to the hands through the repetitive focus and action of the hands, and then gets magnified by observing others with hand pain, and sometimes by being compensated for it.

Edward Siedle, contributing writer at Forbes' Magazine, stated that his shoulder began to hurt after seeing the guy next to him in shoulder pain. A lady wrote to me that her feet began hurting after she saw an advertisement that said flip-flops were bad for the feet. I've had people tell me they got knee pain soon after seeing someone else in knee pain. Others have experienced severe pain after their parents or doctors warned them to be careful to avoid getting a certain pain. Admonitions themselves are guided images that pull the problem to the person through memetic suggestion, magnified by the fear of getting it.

One lady I communicated with experienced severe pain in her feet within 24 hours after her mother told her, "I hope the pain doesn't go to your feet!" And of course, the worst one regarding back pain is when the physician tells the sufferer that his discs are causing his pain—at that point ... the spine becomes the new obsessive focal point for diverting anxiety.

In the rotating hall of mirrors of life, we constantly reflect our strengths and flaws back to us, and to one another. Hence, we're always potential prey to falling for what others emit, as long as we feel the need to be true to them and not to ourselves. We are at further risk if we can't recognize that what is being reflected back is false, or only partly true. Others are also imperfect—hosting their expectations and traits is a flawed process because there's no truth in them for us. The only Truth is *already* inside of us.

Some have said, "Well, the doctors and parents were just smart enough to see the problem coming, and then warn the person!" But the proof that this is not true has always been and will continue to be that the people heal once they suddenly realize they have been memed into the symptom. This is where the phrase "through the looking glass" comes from. Everything is upside down. What we once thought to be real, we now know to be false.

## Repackaging Pain for Profit

Adding to the mass confusion (beyond EPS) is that the labels of pain are changed in order to **segment the problems**, to better market the cures. What was once called carpal tunnel (CT) has been re-labeled as repetitive stress injury (RSI), and again as repetitive stress disorder (RSD). The ole' TMJ, temporomandibular joint disorder has now switched to TMD, temporomandibular joint dysfunction. The currently popular label of fibromyalgia is also being tagged as central sensitization disorder (CSD). What was once called colitis is now dubbed irritable bowel syndrome. What physicians once regularly diagnosed as bursitis is now regularly diagnosed as "rotator cuff tears," or "rotator cuff strains."

On and on it goes: the names periodically change to further narrow down the definitions, so that specialists can claim expertise in the new arena. These particular maladies are not physical body problems, and they are not different things. All of them have been proven to be part of TMS, The Mindbody Syndrome.

There's no logical reason for the confusion. Pain is either the result of a physical structural problem, or it isn't. The body is either failing or it's responding to unconscious activity. And the body rarely fails. The body is strong and resilient. Destructive labels like piriformis syndrome (PS), trigeminal neuralgia (TN), myofascial pain syndrome (MPS), pudendal neuralgia (PN), idiopathic pain syndrome (IPS), plantar fasciitis, fibromyalgia, carpal tunnel, bursitis, painful bladder syndrome (PB), irritable bowel (IBS), and TMD, are effects of emotions. They are not physical body problems, nor are they different things. They are one and the same, and serving the same purpose as back pain. The very segmenting of problems into various classifications is doing widespread harm, and creating epidemics of problems.

However, as Dr. Sarno proved, these symptoms all serve the person as favors to them, by protecting them. And so the sufferers of these new-fangled pain labels tend to defend their specific acronyms with vigor. They do so because the pain provides them with the **safety net they need**—enabling them to cope through their daily stressors and duties, to hide their past, as a crutch. If someone is struggling, they're not going to simply allow someone else to kick their crutches away.

Sufferers who believe their body is defective also begin to identify with their pain, defined by their new pain label. At that point, it becomes much more difficult to help them. Their diversions are the nets on which they can safely fall back, and who doesn't want to feel safe?

One of the newer labels in dealing with low back pain is referred to as **multidisciplinary bio-psycho-social rehabilitation**, or **MBR**. In a recent report on an MBR trial, the study's designers concluded[50]:

> Patients with chronic LBP (low back pain) receiving MBR are likely to experience less pain and disability than those receiving usual care or a physical treatment. MBR also has a positive influence on work status compared to physical treatment. Effects are of a modest magnitude and should be balanced against the time and resource requirements of MBR programs. More intensive interventions were not responsible for effects that were substantially different to those of less intensive interventions. While we were not able to determine if symptom intensity at presentation influenced the likelihood of success, it seems appropriate that only those people with indicators of significant psychosocial impact are referred to MBR.

Translated into English, that means they had trouble seeing much difference between MBR and the normal ways of dealing with back pain. Rheumatology Update reported on this study: "The Cochrane study, which looked at 41 randomized controlled trials involving 6,858 participants, found a **one point difference** between MBR and usual treatments on a 10-point scale for pain"[51]. Because of its slim margin of perceived effectiveness, their main concern was its cost effectiveness.

The good news is that this model begins to look at the stressors in the sufferers' lives (social), and attempts to determine the person's attitude and thinking (psycho) influences on their back pain. Most discouragingly, the MBR model still assumes that the structure of the spine (bio) is involved in the pain, even though the model's advocates admit there's little correlation between spinal imaging and back symptoms. The idea within this model is to use a team of experts in various fields to help "manage back pain,"—much like the multi-approach attempts. If they eventually drop the bio/neuroscience portion of the model they will have made a greater leap forward to where Dr. Sarno is already standing. It will also help to understand that managing pain should never be an option; eliminating it is the goal—unless the goal is to study for study's sake.*

---

*At the end of many studies it says, "Findings from this study highlight the need for more trials."

Currently, in dealing with back pain we've covered:

- **DSA:** Dr. Sarno's approach
- **MDA:** Multidisciplinary approach
- **MIA:** Medical Industry approach
- **MBR:** Multidisciplinary bio-psycho-social rehabilitation

Each time the problem gets diluted through renaming and repackaging, more of the truth gets distorted, and more grant money is requested. Only Dr. Sarno's approach is working effectively, and it's free. Even if the precise mechanism isn't understood by scientists, it still works.

*Shall I refuse my dinner because I do not fully understand the process of digestion?*

Oliver Heaviside, English physicist

There are many other scientific approaches, and hundreds of other back pain trials going on. I've been in contact with several trial researchers to help spread the word of TMS; but once I tell them how I healed, they stop returning emails and phone calls—only the sound of lonely crickets remains. Most have no interest whatsoever in hearing that many of their questions have already been answered. They're blinded by science.

The interesting part is that none of them are ever curious to learn why so many people are healing around the world. As scientists, you would think they would be at least a little bit curious as to why there's been such great success with TMS. But they've treated me in the same manner that Dr. Sarno said he was treated: they simply ignore me. They are determined to jump through the hoops, spend the grant money, and publish the findings. It's a great career—and it keeps them relevant. But in the long run, they're not helping anyone by ignoring what's working so steadily.

Pains from the head to the toes and many other chronic body symptoms, are from the same process and can be healed without surgery, drugs, injections, or therapy. But few people want to hear it, for the reasons I've already discussed; and few understand it because the EPS factors prevent them from seeing the whole picture clearer.

The currently popular pain coping mechanisms are being re-popularized as variations of old problems, as if to claim that the answers are now closer to being solved, and with a deeper under-standing through progressive scientific trial and error. Contrarily, the opposite is happening, we're getting further away from understanding pain because the answer seekers are heavily invested in the business of studying, and not invested enough in finding the solution. By seg-menting, dissecting, and relabeling pains, they've traveled further from the goal of healing and have ignited an explosion of epidemics.

## Contemporary Diversions

What is currently in vogue and acceptable to use is all around. Take a look ... and see what's now popular to use as a diversion, by observing what everyone is currently being diagnosed as having. When I was younger, no one had heard of a thing called fibromyalgia (which longer ago was sometimes called "galloping rheumatism"). Today, there seems to be a fibro-expert on every corner. Did they uncover an unknown problem through hard work and genius, which those before them weren't aware of? Or did they take an old problem, rename it, and then sell it, through genius?

*Eradicate the image of disease from perturbed thought before it has taken tangible shape in conscious thought ... and you prevent the development of disease. This task becomes easy, if you understand that every disease is an error, and has no character or type, except what mortal mind assigns it. By lifting thought above error, or disease, and contending persistently for truth, you destroy error. When we remove disease by addressing the disturbed mind, giving no heed to the body, we prove that thought alone creates suffering.*

Mary Baker Eddy, 1875[52]

By giving a mindbody effect a name such as fibromyalgia, people were able to profit from it, and spread the problem wider through the weapon of fear. Naming it gives it the character and tangible reality needed to pull sufferers in to the treatments. People desire to have answers for their physical symptoms, and they believe much of what their doctors tell them. However, Frederick Wolfe, MD, the lead author of the 1990 paper that set the diagnostic guidelines for fibromyalgia, has reversed his position on fibromyalgia and has stated that he believes fibro is "a physical response to stress, depression, and economic and social anxiety"[53].

*Some of us in those days thought that we had actually identified a disease, which this (fibromyalgia) clearly is not ... to make people ill, to give them an illness, was the wrong thing.*

Frederick Wolfe, MD[54]

Regarding the fibromyalgia diagnosis, Norton Hadler, MD, has stated, "These people live under a cloud ... and the more they seem to be around the medical establishment, the sicker they get."

I invite everyone to go to YouTube and check out "TMS Healing Wall of Victory – The Great Pain Deception." You can see those who were given the fibro diagnosis, and many other false diagnoses, and healed.

The English poet Thomas Gray wrote that "Where ignorance is bliss, 'tis folly to be wise."* This is often true in so many aspects of life, but people also suffer every day from what they don't know, and what they don't care to believe. If their doctor's diagnosis fits with their need to disguise an emotional process as a "disease," then they may accept the incorrect diagnosis, credulously. But there's also the physician who is led by the scientific method, who isn't considering the person and her life problems. Together they kindle fires of suffering based on false beliefs.

**Belief:** *an opinion, a conviction.*

*Thomas Gray poem, "Ode on a Distant Prospect of Eton College," circa 1747.

# 9

# Moving in the Right Direction

## Pain-demonium and Final Transformation

For three decades, I had been so obsessed on my herniated spinal discs, increasing arthritis, crooked spine, bone spurs, and worsening disc-degeneration, that I didn't know there was a way out that was easier. I spent well over a half-million dollars on physical therapy and fools' errands. But my pain remained relentless. When I discovered that my focus on all the healing techniques I had been trying was keeping me in pain, I was in disbelief. But it was ultimately true. The human spine is the strongest part of the body. It isn't weak and frail like the pain industry has led so many to believe. It doesn't need anything done to it—it's much more resilient than we realize. As former back pain sufferer Allison Mains Beardsley reflected on YouTube in June of 2016:

> *I've had chronic low back pain since I was about 18 years old, and now I'm 35 and I have no more back pain (after discovering TMS) and I do all the things I thought I never could do, so thank you for the people out there pioneering this information. Dr. Sarno I'm forever grateful ... It's interesting because I'd studied kinesiology and the company I founded and created was a Pilates based company, (and) both in my Pilates training and my kinesiology training I was taught about how delicate the spine is, so from an institutional level we have it wrong, our spine is not delicate, we're super strong ... there's so much false information out there. ... So after learning this I started to change my beliefs and thoughts, I had instant relief almost. Almost upon learning the information my back pain went away, but it wasn't 100% gone yet, it took about 5 or 6 months and I would say it's 100% gone now. Yaye! ... Just the awareness of this (TMS) information has brought me tremendous healing and growth. I'm now able to enjoy my life pain-free.*[55]

In 2001, I began helping people, full time, to free themselves from pain by teaching them about the cause of their pain. Almost every one of those people was told by their physicians that they needed immediate disc surgery, or steroid injections, or therapy, or rest, or to get stronger, or this and that—but not one of them did. They all healed,

NOT treating their body. However, they had to first become ready to accept that their bodies were okay, and resume all normal physical activity, without fear.

After success in helping, many persuaded me to write a book on the topic, which I did: *The Great Pain Deception: Faulty Medical Advice Is Making Us Worse.* I was particularly honored when Dr. Sarno happily endorsed it because he's the type of man who doesn't normally do that sort of thing. He simply didn't endorse very many publications in his career because he had to deeply believe in the message if he was going to put his name on it. He's the real-deal, clinician, medical doctor—not a marketer.

I've done pain consulting with hundreds of people, including laborers, teachers, doctors, pain scientists, marketers, pro-athletes, musicians, farmers, health coaches, life coaches, coaches-coaches, psychiatrists, psychologists, lawyers, CEOs, and an Oscar-winning actor. What I've learned, I wanted to share with anyone who will listen, who wants to heal. Today the concept is called "paying it forward." Long ago it was stated as, "To whom much is given, much will be asked." Some of the deepest gratification I've ever experienced is to see someone crying with joy once their pain finally resolved. Those who have healed are testimonials to the efficacy of this elegant process. The truth healed them—not me, not numbers, not science, and it began with understanding certain basic concepts, summarized as:

- **Get a Physical Exam:** Make sure there is no dangerous pathological process occurring—take responsibility for your health. Many folks who are now onto TMS and who are beginning to understand what's going on will tell their physicians not to tell them anything about their MRI results unless it's something dangerous. They no longer want to hear about things like "worn" and "torn" or discs and arthritis. They've begun permanently healing at that point.

- **Take Your Physical Exam Results with a Grain of Salt:** If you decide to hear your exam results that reveal only herniated discs, arthritis as seen on the x-ray, osteophytes (spurs), a crooked spine, spinal narrowing (stenosis), or any other normal change, then be of great cheer! These physical states don't cause back pain, unless in very extreme cases. Experience has shown that they're simply there—almost everyone has these anatomical changes, with or without pain. Pain is the effect of oxygen reduction. Whether the pain is in the limbs, or spine, or any other area, it rarely ever comes from the body's structure.

    ✓ Remember, this doesn't include injuries. But TMS can sneak in after an injury to fool the person into thinking the injury itself is not healing.

- **Reject the Multidisciplinary Approach:** Reject the approach of throwing various techniques at the problem. Attempting multiple techniques basically means, "We don't have a clue what to do, so let's try this and that, and cross our fingers." These techniques include acupuncture, spinal manipulations, core aligning, surgery, injections, core strengthening, losing weight, etc. These approaches are almost always followed by temporary symptom easing, and can paradoxically keep you in pain. The multi-approach is a major factor in the rising pain epidemics, of all sorts. One of the more damaging statements being proclaimed by the industry today is, "One size does not fit all." The more accurate statement should be, "One belief does not fit all." One technique works for one person and not for another because one deeply believed in the technique, but the other did not.

- **Beware of Faulty Diagnoses:** The myth of herniated discs causing pain was exposed decades ago by the greatest pain doctor America has ever known. Surgeons are just now beginning to realize this, as some of them have healed with his work. You cannot pinch a nerve or paralysis will quickly follow, and the pain will stop. A dead nerve cannot transmit pain signals. You also cannot "throw your back out." Spinal discs are strongly attached on both sides of the spine; they cannot slip in and out of place.

    You don't have to strengthen your body's core to heal, and scoliosis does not cause pain. People have scoliosis their entire lives, and then suddenly, as adults, when they experience back pain it's blamed on the curvature.

- **Understand the Reason for Your Pain:** Almost all chronic pain is a diversion by the brain to rivet the sufferer's attention to his body. When powerful emotions hit a certain threshold, the brain reduces blood/oxygen flow to a body area to create a diversion—as a favor— to avoid any emotional pain. The pain is never imagined or faked; it's very real, and extremely painful. Back pain can be viewed as a **best friend** that is trying to both help you and protect you at the same time. It's trying to tell you something very personal and truthful that you don't want to hear, that other people are afraid to tell you. Sometimes the pain is the only thing you can count on.

- **Look at What's Going on in Your Life:** Almost everyone is able to trace their pain back to an event, or a life plateau. Is your marriage in trouble? Does your job stress you out? Did a loved one die or is

someone sick? Did you recently retire? Do you have the Type-T*
"pain personality" of perfectionism, trying to please everyone? Do
you show little emotion? Did you feel emotionally abandoned or
supported as a child? Are you hyper-responsible, a worrier? Are you
an individual driven to win, or succeed? Did you just hit a
milestone age? Are you bored? Are you a catastrophizer? Does your
mind race? What is it that you are not reacting to? Connect your
dots to your pain, and heal. The knowledge of what is occurring—
and acceptance of it at the unconscious level—has tremendous
healing power because once the seal is broken on the brain's
strategy, the pain no longer works as a covert diversion.

- **Try to Understand Why You Need to Believe You Have a Bad
  Back:** When told there is a way to heal their pain forever, many will
  say, "No! My pain is real!" Well, the pain is always real. The more
  important question is, when someone is told they can be relieved
  from their suffering, why isn't their very first question about how to
  do it? Why would anyone fight healing, especially since it requires
  nothing but learning? This is critical in understanding the brain's
  purpose in creating the pain. Of course he wants to believe he has a
  structural problem. That's his brain's intent! Who doesn't listen to
  their brain? But we should instead be listening to our intuition,
  such as in, "Hey, there are millions of people around the world
  healing with Dr. Sarno's information. Is my spine worse than all of
  theirs? Nothing I have ever tried has worked for me." What does
  your intuition tell you? That you have the most unique spine in the
  world, or that maybe you have TMS?

Some sufferers react with extreme hate, and occasional violence, at
the notion that there's nothing wrong with their spine. They spit, point
angry fingers, throw things, and stomp out of the room, knocking
things over in fits of rage. These actions are strong indicators they have
TMS. *The closer to the fire the more it burns.* They only hear, "Your pain
is not real." But no one is saying that. The truth about their pain is
threatening to expose their brain's purpose, so it must be strongly
rejected, like holy water. It's easier to believe in a failing spine than
admit to a life that has not gone as planned. One of the most common
questions people ask me is why their friends and relatives don't believe
them about TMS. I often read emails like, "My wife (or husband) won't
talk to me any more after I suggested she (or he) has TMS." The same is

*The Type T is a high-tension personality. It is perfectionistic, conscientious,
goodist, gentle, kind, driven, and a detail-oriented worrier. Not all sufferers fit
into all of these categories, but these are the most common attributes of the
pain personality.

true for relatives, neighbors, bosses, friends, and co-workers. Almost everyone is furious if it is suggested they may not have a broken body. One would think this would be great news! But it isn't welcomed.

By rejecting that their symptoms are created by internal forces, they fall faithfully into their brain's ingenious strategy of deceit, and their suffering continues. And one of the most common misconceptions people have is that TMS is for everyone else but them.

I've also experienced another phenomenon in which the sufferer will reject the notion of TMS, but silently go buy the books, read about it, and get better. Then, once healed, they claim that they were cured by their last spinal adjustment, or a new type of exercise, or gimmick. Their ego wouldn't allow them to admit to TMS openly (due to shame), but they knew it was true and wanted to heal on their own terms (placating ego). In this way, they can still refute TMS as being true.

I have literally heard it hundreds of times, the most common of the responses, "That's all definitely true, but my back pain is real." The reason they can't understand that they, too, have TMS is that their doctor told them they have a problem.

- The pain begins with the sufferer.
- The problems begin with the doctor, followed by the need for the sufferer to believe he has a structural problem, and ends with his belief in his doctor.

In the effort to out-heal Mother Nature, pain practitioners have become the leading cause of epidemics, from fibromyalgia to chronic fatigue. The truth in healing is up against a multi-trillion dollar juggernaut called the "medical industry" that is hell-bent on treating symptoms. The true message of "how to heal" gets blocked at every turn by people inside the industry who profit from the treating; and by publications that depend on advertisement dollars from the industry. When the few articles on TMS are published in magazines, they're always surrounded by advertisements, above or below, and from the left and right, with ads by laser surgery groups, drug companies, or mattress companies, preying on what people don't know.

We currently have available the most advanced equipment and medical techniques ever possessed by humankind, and yet pain epidemics are widespread. If a sufferer visits a practitioner for pain, whether it's in the hands and feet, knees or shoulders, or neck or back, **the physician will find something** on the imaging to blame it on. The doctors should be screening for danger only, and then talking to the sufferer about her life problems, and her history. Less is more. In the case of TMS, no treatment is everything.

> *This is important in medicine. It's all so universal, and it's*
> *important to make the right diagnosis. If you make the wrong*
> *diagnosis, if you attribute the pain to something structural, or*
> *if you say, "The reflux is due to your stomach acting up and*
> *you have to take this drug or that drug," then people will*
> *continue to have symptoms. This is why the back pain*
> *problem is of epidemic proportions in the United States.*
>
> John E. Sarno, MD[5]

Modern medicine is good. It has saved the lives of millions of people, and helped to improve the quality of countless others. I am a strong advocate for new procedures and higher learning. However, regarding **The Mindbody Syndrome**, the use of these medical advancements is literally hurting people.

## TMS: The Man Sarno

John Sarno is an international treasure. He helped to heal Howard Stern, isn't that enough? No?? How about others he's helped? They include radio host Don Imus, PGA golfer Ben Crane, the late great Anne Bancroft, filmmaker Michael Galinksy, Seinfeld creator Larry David, Forbes' writer/contributor Ed Siedle, former Senator Tom Harkin, television host Greg Gutfeld, writer/producer Jonathan Ames, pioneering direct marketer Marty Edelston, comedian/writer Janette Barber, journalist John Stossel, US Secretaries of State, acclaimed writers and actors, high level athletes including Olympians, musicians of all levels, general medical practitioners, pain specialists, soldiers, Marines, construction workers, firemen, marketers, entrepreneurs, chiropractors, engineers, teachers, accountants, singers, nurses, photographers, writers, language translators, surgeons, oncologists, loggers, joggers, bloggers, and people who drink lagers—sufferers from every walk of life. He has eased the suffering of legions of open-minded people, including yours truly. After 50 years in medicine he established himself as America's best doctor. Isn't that enough? Apparently not. People still demand spurious numbers for unnecessary proof.

I receive emails about Dr. Sarno from Nantucket to Norway, Canada to Korea, Jersey to Germany, Frisco to France, and from the Balkans to the Kiwi-lands down under. When I do coaching and consultations the folks will often hold up his books that have been translated into their primary languages such as German, Italian, or Spanish. His work is being disseminated internationally as more people heal across the globe with his medical observations, and his praiseworthy courage.

Dozens of books are coming out from people he helped, telling their stories, as well as new TMS-healing websites, YouTube videos, Facebook pages, and the Peer Review Network TMSWiki.org. People he helped to heal are now shouting for joy from the mountaintops to the Internet. He's affectionately known by all as "the good doctor." But he has been so much more; not only is he a great doctor, he's a great man.

Despite all of his great successes, Dr. Sarno was pushed out of teaching at NYU, and eventually stopped eating in the cafeteria with the other doctors due to the cold shoulders from his peers (different from "frozen shoulder," which is TMS). Why has he been treated this way? Because he is helping to ease the suffering of people by telling them they didn't need surgery, drugs, injections, or physical therapy. He's persona non grata to many within the pain industry because he didn't play along, and a pariah to many laymen because he didn't tell them what they wanted to hear. He simply wanted to help. History will judge his career, but for those of us whose lives he saved, we only have thanks, adoration, respect, and love for him.

## The Great Pain Deception

The operative word in my first book's title is "Deception." That word was heavily ruminated on for about a month, and chosen for three main reasons.

- First, the most obvious reason is that pain is a deception by the brain to convince the sufferer that he or she is physically wounded.

- Second, a small number within the medical industry know that what they're doing isn't working, but they keep on doing it.

- Third is a concept of "self-deception." Self-deception means that you have convinced yourself that the lie is the truth. People in hated jobs and draining relationships will smile and pretend that life is good (a reaction-formation, discussed soon). But they break down crying when reaching a little deeper into their pain. People are rarely who they're pretending to be. Once that massive river of repression begins to flow, a healing catharsis begins. In the interim, their pain is forever present to assist them in the deception that something is actually wrong with their spine. They **cannot heal** until they stop deceiving themselves.

The subtitle of my first book is "Faulty Medical Advice Is Making Us Worse." Since TMS pain emanates from his brain's fervent desire to convince him that his body is broken, all medical advice that points to his body as being the problem only assists his brain with the deception, making his problem worse. He must stop all forms of treatment, or he prolongs his suffering. Here's just one example:

Marc D. Sopher, MD, a TMS physician who trained under Dr. Sarno, had a patient who had been in pain for eight years, with perineal pain. The man couldn't walk, sit, or stand without pain. He had seen several doctors, and had tried many treatments. In desperation, he made a visit to Dr. Sopher. He was scheduled the very next week to have a spinal cord stimulator implanted, on the advice of his physician. Fortunately, he went to see Dr. Sopher first, who examined him and concluded that his pain was from TMS. Within three weeks the man was doing much better, within three months he had dramatically improved and was living a normal life again.

Through eight years and all of his doctor visits, his medical treatments were making him worse. Once he realized, and accepted, that his body was okay, and that he was reacting to unconscious emotions, he healed. This is "knowledge therapy" because his new awareness that his brain was trying to deceive him had initiated healing.

> *When I teach people what this is all about, what's going on physically, and what's going on psychologically, I think the rage is no longer as threatening as it was before, and so they don't need to have symptoms.*
>
> John E. Sarno, MD[5]

## The Pain Personality

Personality is the most important ingredient in creating tension in the body. Understanding how the sufferer thinks and functions is, therefore, the most important aspect in helping them heal. Everyone has TMS to varying degrees, but most don't know it because they're fixated on their body's sensations. The perfectionist, however, will deny emotions in order to forge ahead. Perfection, used as a means of avoiding rejection creates great health-damaging tension. So it's germane to ask, "Is it better to be perfect, or happy?" Why do we treat our bodies so neglectfully, avoiding our own needs, trying to keep everyone else happy? The deeper understanding of those questions often leads to healing.

TMS shows up in endless forms that most would consider normal body problems, such as stomach problems, chronic sleep issues, skin distress, depression and anxiety, vision concerns, infections, vertigo, nausea, ringing in the ears, heart symptoms, and immune problems, etc. We can't express all of our concerns at all times because we aren't aware of many powerful forces within us, due to **repression:** a primary survival tool.

**Repressing:** *expelling thoughts, memories, and emotions into the unconscious.*

Repression is a powerful mechanism for survival by enabling us to perform our duties of interacting with others, while hiding certain aspects of ourselves from them that we deem to be unacceptable to them, and so to us as well. Repression enables us to cast from our consciousness those events that threaten our persona, as well as, those things that are about to overwhelm us. It helps us to live with others, to function under threat of danger. The danger can be life-threatening, or a social danger such as shame. Repression can be viewed as moving our incoming sensory information from the present moment into the body, which acts as a holding cell for the rejected information. But that rejected information still exists in the body even when the individual is not aware of it. It's simply been shunned and sent to the unconscious, which is the body. In everyone with TMS, they've abused the tool of repression by ignoring specifically important thoughts and emotions that mean very much to them. Repression has gone awry, due to a perfectionistic and stoic personality.

At some point, repression reaches an unsustainable limit, and the threat of emotions flowing back into consciousness begins to disrupt **autonomic functions**—demanding to be expressed, and yet denied by ego. The more repressive the tendencies (Type-T personality), the more unaware the sufferers are of specific thoughts and emotions, acting like human robots, going through the motions—living in a frozen emotional state. The end result is great pain and poor health because they're not listening to the whispering voices inside them (the symptoms). If they felt all their emotions there would be no need for back pain; but humans are not currently wired to react any other way.

  Pain is a direct result of personality, not genetics.

Her inability to express herself and her lack of awareness of how she truly feels is causing her pain because she cannot express, or will not express, or doesn't know how to express herself. As a child, she was not allowed to express her fear and anger, or she never had the opportunity. Now she's an adult who never learned how to sense, and then release her emotions of anger, and sorrow, and frustration. She screens her life through her **corrupted memory**, feeling that she is who she's pretending to be, thinking that she's living "perfectly."

Many children are taught that it's bad to be angry and that they should be ashamed, and silent. The result is a child-adult who never developed a means to feel from the heart. They can intellectually describe their pain, such as, "sharp, buzzing, deep, burning, etc.," but they have trouble explaining what it's telling them. The sharp back pain is her way of **somaticizing**, which means that her undeveloped self is expressing itself through her body, the only way it knows how.

## TMS is a Tough Mother to Sell: Resistance to Change

In the words of former back pain sufferer Howard Stern, regarding Dr. Sarno's work, "I beg anyone who is seeking a solution to pain to study the amazing and revolutionary approach outlined here. I did, and it changed my life." Howard is not alone in his zeal to help others. I can't think of a single person who has healed from back pain, who hasn't immediately said, "I wanted to help everyone I knew, but my family and friends think I'm crazy." As soon as they heal, they're so overjoyed that they want to tell everyone whom they love, and to share in the happiness of being pain-free. But the message falls on deaf ears, past rolling eyeballs, over mocking lips, and into the teeth of sarcasm.

Now we're nudging ever closer to the ultimate cause of pain: **resistance**. The Sufi philosopher Rumi wrote, "Why do you stay in prison when the door is so wide open?" The essence of Rumi's question will soon answer itself, if you follow the logic all the way through. At that point, your healing has begun. Back pain has to be learned away, it cannot be doctored away. Trying to medicalize the spine into being pain-free is like picking up mercury. You can chase its elusiveness around forever.

As I stated earlier, the confusion over back pain comes from EPS; the three intertwining components of *ego*, *placebo*, and the *shifting symptoms*. The reasons for confusion remain clear—**ego** contrives emotional blind spots to protect the lies; **placebos** temporarily please; and the **shifting symptoms** provide cover by ostensibly appearing to have solved the earlier problem.

Why there is confusion is easy to see—but why is there so much **resistance** to a proven healing message? The short answer is that the addict needs the needle.

If a person can't face certain aspects of himself, and his pain exists to hide those aspects, then why would that person want his pain to go away? He may find any excuse to *protect his pain's purpose,* even if he has to deny something that can help him. The more painful the emotion being hidden, in the form of back pain, the more convinced he is that his pain is caused by his spine, and the more likely his pain is not caused by his spine. The brain has a perfect scheme going on.

Another major reason for resistance is that sufferers truly want to believe in their physician. This is natural in every society. When people are sick, and scared of death and dying, they turn to their healer as a last line of defense. Frightened people naturally look up to their doctors, and tend to heed their words. They make the desperate error of believing that everything their doctor tells them is true.

Yet another reason for resistance is that many view psychologically-induced pain as a weakness, when it is not. It is in fact, a great strength to not act out in aggression, to stand up to responsibilities, and to try to be a good person. These are often the strongest and most talented people in society: in pain, yet acting on their duties. The father in pain getting up to go to work each day, the mother pushing through her career and school, taking care of her family—despite her pain.

Having chronic pain does not indicate a mental disorder. In fact, these people cope too well. They're "too sane" in the sense that they can't lighten up and let go of some order and control. Karl Menninger, MD, founder of the renowned Menninger Clinic in Topeka, Kansas, noted that psychotic patients "as a rule enjoy the most robust health"—and when the psychosis begins to wane, the physical health problems return. Back pain sufferers are mentally okay. They may approach neurosis at times, but they're sane. They need to have more fun, let more go, stop obsessing on their spine, stop trying to heal, become more active, get silly, and find a life passion—get a little crazy. They also need to find a path that takes them where they know they want to be, which is where their pain is pushing them. They need to open themselves to change.

Finally of course, the primary cause of resistance is that the cause of back pain is outside of awareness. People have trouble believing what they can't see, relying on intellect (proof), rather than intuition (a feeling with a choice). Education of what's going on between mind and body is paramount to healing, and to a better life. Healing comes from learning, and learning comes from education, or experience. Intelligence comes in many forms but its intellectual problem-solving characteristic is its biggest hindrance to healing. Truth heals, but our gut feeling brings us to the classroom. The heart knows the way and is open, but the head often resists. What does your gut tell you about TMS? Are the millions who have healed all wrong, exceptions? Or is it true?

*The voice of the intelligence is drowned out by the roar of fear. It is ignored by the voice of desire. It is contradicted by the voice of shame. It is biased by hate and extinguished by anger. Most of all it is silenced by ignorance.*

Karl A. Menninger, MD

## Confusion and Resistance Summarized Together:

- **Ego:** Sees TMS as a weakness, hides aspects of Self, and thinks the current understanding is the only way.

- **Sufferers' vested interest in not healing:** Some are compensated to stay away from despised jobs. They go golfing or fishing on disability pay instead of to a miserable job. Others are "leaders of their cause," such as regional or national fibromyalgia, RSD, or "fatigue awareness" directors, who have fought hard for grant money, for studies. Some of them have little patience for a mindbody solution that would rob them of their passion and purpose, and of their professional goals.

- **The brain's protective mechanism:** The pain exists to protect the sufferer from dangerous emotions. If the pain was to leave, they would be faced with an imperfect image of themselves. Anything that threatens to take away that barrier must be rebuffed.

- **The process is unconscious:** The sufferer doesn't know it's occurring.

- **The belief that emotional pain is a weakness:** It isn't.

- **Belief in their doctors:** Even when their doctor is wrong.

- **Correlation errors:** Imaging tests show "problems" at the site of the pain, resulting in spurious correlations.

- **Rejection because TMS healing is too simplistic:** A common reaction is, "You're trying to take something that's very complex (healing) and make it too simple (with TMS)." But it's just the opposite. "The industry" is trying to take something very simple and keep it complex.

- **Placebo effects:** Fool people into believing that they indeed "had something wrong" that was somehow fixed.

- **Symptom Imperative shift:** Makes people feel that the last procedure worked in them. But it only changed into a new problem.

- **Conviction that the pain feels structural:** The pain feels so musculoskeletal that the sufferer links what he sees on his imaging to his sharp pain: creating a straw man, holding a red herring, choking on a smokescreen of confusion.

- **Admonition that Dr. Sarno took people to "the cure" too quickly:** I occasionally talk to practitioners, and pain advocate groups, some of whom feel Dr. Sarno "may have found" the answer, but they still want to jump through the hoops, one at a time, not wanting to see the end yet. Some have bluntly said, "I've worked for years to get the funding for my grant; I'm not gonna blow it now."

They prefer to do the testing, walk through the studies, write the books, and make the money, in order to have a good career and life for their families, as justified compensation for years of dedication to their cause. They don't necessarily refute TMS healing, but it's an inconvenience for them right now.

If Dr. Sarno's work was to be taken seriously, there would be economic chaos within the medical industry. So it must either get rejected, or at a minimum, parsed into smaller pieces, and delayed until post-retirement.

I've also spoken to a handful of people who have spent years trying to qualify for disability for their back pain. They've invested time and money seeking to be paid for time off, or compensated for work lost. Their hopes pinned on compensation they feel will help them avoid even more pain. And these folks need to be taken very seriously. Some have committed suicide after being ruled fit to work following their application for disability benefits[56].

## A Man Without a Country

Pain is a warning signal. In every situation it shields against potential danger. In the case of acute structural injury or disease it warns us that the body is under threat. But in the case of TMS, the brain creates (and recreates) the pain for the purpose of protecting the individual from emotions that are too sad, too powerful, or too threatening. When the pain is unknowingly self-created in this manner it is shielding the sufferer from emotional danger; it is, therefore, often protected by that sufferer in many ways, one of which is by vehemently denying that TMS is true. Delivering the TMS message then becomes an art form—a delicate balancing act between helping, and not harming.

On occasion people engaged in various alternative health fields will contact me to say, "I'm with ya man! Screw the medical industry, it's hurting us!" I have to then politely tell them that I'm telling everyone to stop what they, too, are advocating: all the alternative health stuff. There's never been a reply at that point.

I was invited to speak in Fort Lauderdale, Florida in front of 16,000 people at some type of alternative health summit. The organizers read my book and told me I would be a "perfect fit to speak." When I looked at the other guest speakers I could see that I was advocating against every one of them. So I asked the organizers, "You do realize that I'm going to stand up there and tell the audience to not listen to any of your other guest speakers?" I never heard anything back from them, except a car door slamming and tires peeling out. It's a money-driven "do something to the body" industry because that's where the livings are made. And everyone feels they have the correct answer. The cure for most of our health problems is to do nothing except to find balance; diminish ego consciousness—and open the third eye.

There are, of course, serious states of health that require some medical intervention. This cannot be overstated. Be careful! But it's equally important to understand why those disorders form, and why they become so serious.

Stephen Flynn, a chiropractor practicing in Maine, who recovered from stage four metastatic cancer wrote to me the following:

> Facing death at the age of twenty-five creates an urgency from within that cannot be easily put into words. Why is cancer so difficult to explain? It may seem like a shallow question to ask, but the examination of it gnawingly repeats itself and spreads outward like a virus, to family and friends.
>
> To calm my mind, I used a variety of mind body techniques, conventional medicine and good reliable research, all of which kept and keep me alive today. Long before I read about the power of the mind, I experienced its tremendous force. Because I had this experience I lent considerable credence to my own participation in defeating my disease. However, your book The Great Pain Deception taught me to look at my own participation in causing the expression of my cancer. Alas, you gave me the answer as to "why" it's so difficult to explain. The awareness I gained from facing my own imminent death and then applying it back to my life at the time of diagnosis clearly demonstrated to me where the true disease was rooted and now no longer lives. My cancer was caused by me and my self-derived emotional dissonance. My unconscious mind created a formidable disparity between who I thought I was and wanted to be, and the ultimate truth of self. The dysfunction was rooted in a myriad of multifaceted and repressed internal conflicts that lingered and remained unresolved.
>
> I strived so hard to provide comfort and ease to the people around and close to me, to keep them all happy. The harder I tried, the more I wore down, the more I became unaware of what I was doing to myself. I cannot express this enough ever since reading your book (GPD) I see the world ... the whole world, differently. Truly the most fascinating work I have experienced. [Reprinted with permission]

Doctor Flynn's compelling story is a true inspiration that ignites the fires of hope in everyone. We unconsciously contribute to our own health problems more than we fully understand. Steve's journey back into balance is a powerful example of healing that required some modern medical attention, mindbody practice, deepening awareness, and courage. The life must be protected from danger first. Regarding most back pain, however, the common structural states are not diseases: they're natural occurrences. So it's important to realize that there's a world of difference between certain health issues and others. Some conditions require exigent medical treatment, most do not. Regarding back pain, it's been proven time and time again that it's critical to stop treating the spine.

Trying to explain, to spinal pain sufferers, the difference between conditions that need medical intervention and those that do not is precarious work. There are almost no allies in the "do nothing" view of healing. The message is surreal to most because we've all been taught that our bodies need never-ending repair. Health is big business. And to keep that business ongoing, many myths have morphed into accepted facts.

## Back Pain Myths

- **Herniated discs are pinching nerves:** They are not. The most commonly accepted myth regarding back pain is that it's caused by bulging discs. Dr. Sarno proved decades ago that structural changes are normal byproducts of aging—"grey hairs of the spine." As he noted, "... the idea that they (nerves) are being pinched is usually fantasy and, once again, there is much ado about nothing."

- **The spine is weak:** It is not.

- **Spinal discs slip in and out:** They cannot.

- **Scoliosis causes back pain:** It does not.

- **Back Pain Is From Normal Aging:** The proof that back pain is not caused simply by getting older is that older folks in their 70s and 80s heal regularly once they accept that their pain is not from their aged spine.

- **The spine is too damaged to heal:** I was told that my spine was "too far gone" to heal, so bad that it couldn't even be manipulated ever again. I've also been contacted by several people who healed after they were told that their spines "looked like mush," and had "extensive degeneration." No matter how many surgeries you've had, or how long you've suffered, or how much your doctor doesn't know, you can heal if you have TMS.

- **Sitting or lifting is bad for the back:** Sitting is completely harmless to the spine. However, when pain ensues from sitting, an "association error" begins—like Pavlov feeding his hounds; pain then occurs each time while sitting. Lifting and moving dramatically increase spine health, and build confidence for healing.

- **Scar tissue slows healing:** It does not. However, if the sufferer is told that scarring slows healing then it might, if she believes it. Dr. Sarno never saw scar tissue inhibit healing, and neither have the TMS physicians I've spoken to.

- **You must journal to heal:** You do not. I never journaled, and I went 10 years before I met anyone who had to journal to heal. Journaling can work, and has helped a number of people, but it isn't always necessary in healing.
- **Mindbody back pain is a neurological disorder:** It is not. It is a temporary strategy by the brain to help the individual cope.

Those are the **major myths**, but there are countless other minor myths regarding the causes of back pain floating around in the back pain world, landing where they may, adding to the mountainous mess, such as:

- Kids' backpacks carried on one shoulder;
- Sitting wrong, or on wrong chairs (poor ergonomics);
- Poor i-posture;
- Low iron count;
- Cracked vertebrae from years ago that wasn't diagnosed in time;
- Poor computer workstation "habits";
- Low waist jeans;
- Typing over a keyboard;
- Smoking;
- Bending other than with your knees only;
- Wrong types of shoes;
- Soft beds;
- Poor sleeping habits;
- Getting in and out of bed wrong;
- Your pain is all in your mind;
- Etc. ... the misunderstanding is endless. As long as the cause is searched for on the outside, the pains will continue on the inside. Pain practitioners simply make up explanations out of thin air, which adds to the problem if the sufferer needs a diversion and begins to worry about the new red herring. Bad advice has gotten us to pandemic stages; more bad advice cannot get us out.

*A new type of thinking is essential if mankind is to survive and move to higher levels.*

Albert Einstein, PhD[57]

# 10

# From Problem to Epidemic

Problems elevate from simple problems to epidemics when:

- Physicians validate problems as being physical (body failing).
  - ✓ **Sanctioning through codifying**
- Society concedes that a particular pain diversion is acceptable by setting up systems to "help victims."
  - ✓ **Compensating through pleasing**
- Support groups form to help sufferers with symptoms.
  - ✓ **Multiplying through reinforcing**

## Norwegian Necks

As a scientist, Norwegian neurologist, Harald Shrader, MD, was curious to know why there was an explosion of whiplash cases in his tiny country of Norway: a country of 70,000 chronic whiplash sufferers, and only 4.2 million people.[*]

Out of scientific curiosity, Shrader led a team to Lithuania to see what was going on there because Lithuania had little to no awareness of whiplash, and no system of compensation for it. Upon arrival, Shrader and his colleagues began to question Lithuanian drivers who had been in rear-end collisions; and they set up a control group for a study on whiplash. The end result as Shrader concluded was: "No one in the study group had disabling or persistent symptoms as a result of the car accident."

Not a single person in the Lithuanian study experienced the effects of whiplash after being hit in a rear-end collision. The Lithuanians even had trouble understanding the concept, and were amazed that anyone could possibly feel the effects of an accident that happened over a year ago.

Both Norway and Lithuania had similar populations and a similar number of car accidents. Remarkably, most Lithuanians had never even heard of whiplash. They also didn't sue each other for compensation, so there was no money to be gained in accidents, and most medical bills were paid by the Lithuanian government, so no money came out of the pockets of those involved in car accidents.

---

[*]Remember, the neck is the upper back.

Here's the main point: it's not that the people in Norway weren't in terrible pain, or were faking their symptoms. Their pain was real; but they were lured into thinking there would be lingering symptoms and long drawn-out expensive healing times because their country's system was set up to accommodate the problem. The doctors in Norway were telling people after the rear-end collisions to be careful, to rest their neck, brace their neck, and to anticipate long-term pain—to **expect it**. The doctors in Lithuania were telling people after rear-end collisions to go home, go back to work.

Norway created a perfect atmosphere for an epidemic storm:

- **Sanctioning:** Norwegian physicians and citizens bought into the notion of lingering neck pain.

- **Compensating:** Norway had an elaborate system for compensating victims of whiplash.

- **Multiplying:** Norwegians observed one another in pain; unconsciously spreading it by making it acceptable to have.

Norwegians expected pain: *epidemic.*
Lithuanians had no expectations of pain: *no epidemic.*

## Forest for the Trees

I suppose a study could be contorted to show how strong Lithuanian's necks are compared to Norwegian necks. No doubt someone could profit from studying their neck differences. But until then, a blind man with a cane can see the distinction between the two countries: yet some folks look at this scenario and say, "It's not true." The blind person needs a cane like a skeptic needs a number. They both rely on their devices because they can't see any further than the information it sends back.

Accommodating pain invites it to linger. The Norwegians, seeing pain all around them, "absorbed it"—and so it thrived. Each victim infected the next through unconscious suggestion (meme selection)—perpetuating, reflecting, and magnifying the error. The mind is that powerful. It will adapt to the current circumstance using what it sees in order to fit in, adapt, cope, survive, **to connect**. If you tell a person they are a victim for long enough even they will begin to believe it.

## Hands Across America

In the United States, there was a 467 percent increase in the number of people claiming disability for carpal tunnel syndrome between 1989 and 1994[58]. In 1994 alone, 849,000 *new cases* of carpal tunnel syndrome occurred, according to the National Center for Health

Statistics. Is it possible that nearly a million pairs of hands suddenly fell apart between 1989 and 1994?

The carpal tunnel, hip, shoulder, fibro, chronic fatigue, knee, feet, hand, and back pain epidemics are a direct result of the need for the diversions, fueled by the passing along of the symptoms through memetic observation—magnified by systems set up to accommodate, and to compensate *victims*. The symptoms and pains are all real; the brain is simply capitalizing on the opportunity of the day when it needs help coping.

In an interview with Reuters Health, Russell Gelfman, MD, from the Mayo Clinic in Rochester, Minnesota stated that the increase in carpal tunnel, "… was quite rapid in the 1980s and it would be difficult to attribute the causes for it solely to changes in medical or physical risk factors … we believe that increased awareness by the public, in particular the publicity resulting from the epidemic of work-related carpal tunnel syndrome, may explain some of the trend."

> *I think that prior to around 1985 or so there are really very few cases of carpal tunnel syndrome that are paid for out of workers' compensation. And then you see this big growth between 1985 and about 1995 where many more cases are claimed as work-related. And this is the so-called epidemic of carpal tunnel syndrome that got people quite interested in and **focused** on CTS (carpal tunnel syndrome) in the late 80s early 90s.*
>
> Bradley A. Evanoff, MD, MPH[59],
> occupational health and safety researcher

However, just as quickly as the carpal-trend heated up it cooled down. In 2006, carpal cases tumbled by 21%, and the number of cases fell by half between 2005 and 2006 among workers in professional and business services[60]. So, did the hands and wrists suddenly become healthier again? Or was the epidemic amplified by observation and compensation, and suddenly replaced by another diversionary fad?

Edward V. Craig, MD, stated in the commentary for an NBC article entitled "What ever happened to carpal tunnel? Trendy techno malady has eased, but we've already got a new ache," that "Putting a name to what is essentially an overuse problem leads the patient to believe there is serious injury, giving the condition a magnitude often undeserved, rather than recognizing it as one of the aches periodically experienced by each of us"[61].

The same may be said for hip pain, and many other in-vogue health diversions that suddenly appear, and then fade (shift to a new physical area), when a newer more popularly acceptable coping mechanism rises to awareness, and is sanctioned by the medical business as a "legitimate problem." Hip replacement surgery in the US, for people aged 45 and over, increased 45 percent from 2000-2010[62]. Some industry supporters claim that the increases are due to getting better at such techniques. But we know that many of these people heal once they discover TMS. And that after hip surgery, the brain will simply shift its target elsewhere, if the psychological circumstances still warrant a distraction. Physicians and sufferers aren't aware of the Symptom Imperative. The surgical techniques most likely aren't doing anything beyond placebo, in the majority of the cases.

> *Jack was a former athlete, now in his 40s, with left hip pain. His orthopedist told him that he would benefit from a new hip joint as his x-ray showed 'significant' degenerative changes. After this visit his left hip pain increased and he mentioned it to me at the time of his annual physical exam. When he told me that his right hip felt fine, I asked him to humor me by having both of his hips x-rayed. On x-ray, both hips had the same 'degenerative' changes, yet his right hip did not hurt! I advised him to put off surgery, resume activity and not pay too much attention to his hips. Following these instructions, his discomfort subsided and he successfully resumed exercise and athletics.*
>
> Marc D. Sopher, MD[63]

## Initiating and Perpetuating Suffering

It can't be overstated that it's the doctors who are among the main magnifiers of pain and continue to be, every day. Sometimes they **initiate** the symptoms by pointing to harmless changes in the body as potential problems, like herniated discs, (osteo) arthritis, one leg being longer than the other, etc., increasing the individual's awareness, obsession, anxiety, fear, and therefore tension. There may have been no problem at that point; but now the worrying individual begins to shift awareness, and a new problem begins.

However, more commonly than initiating the problem, the **physicians perpetuate the suffering,** through poor diagnoses. In the case of TMS, the sufferer comes into the office complaining of pain, and the doctor confirms that the pain is coming from the structural body. The sufferer, if she accepts this, suffers chronically as a result of a faulty confirmation.

In the first instance the doctor created the fear. The individual then goes home, thinks about "the new problem" and symptoms begin to appear. In the second instance, the more common case, the patient comes to the doctor with a symptom; and the doctor, feeling inclined to come up with an answer, mistakenly correlates natural body changes with the pain. Both cases are *diagnosing nocebo effects.*\* The diagnosis harms the person. Lamentably, there was often nothing wrong to begin with, and a spurious correlation is formed between what was seen on imaging (as a natural occurrence), to the sensations described by the sufferer.

## Abby Normal

TMS mindbody and life coach Abigail Steidley learned along the same hard road that many others have traveled. In her 20s, she suffered from intense pelvic pain syndromes. The following is an interaction she had with her physician during a physical examination:

> **Her physician:** (Snapping the rubber gloves off ... the doctor popped his head up) *Your pelvic floor is a disaster. You have pelvic floor dysfunction, vulvodynia, vulvar vestibulitis, and vulvar dysesthesia.*
>
> **Abigail:** *Why did I get these syndromes?*
>
> **Her physician:** *We don't really know why they occur.*

Abigail then told him that she was depressed, and anxious. But he didn't appear to be concerned or able, to correlate her pain to the emotions that she was describing to him. He was determined to "doctor her problem away" as taught to him in medical school. Abigail had been hanging all her hopes on that one appointment, "... as if simply walking through the door would bring relief." But she left more depressed and disappointed.

She had suffered through years of interstitial cystitis and vaginal pain. She had trouble sitting, walking, wearing underwear or jeans, or doing anything that involved movement. She was lost and hopeless. Alone. However, when the student is ready, the teacher will appear. A friend gave her Dr. Sarno's book, *The Mindbody Prescription*. She saw herself inside its pages and implemented the good doctor's ideas into her life. Sure enough, her pain and other symptoms, such as burning, itching, numbness, etc., faded away.

Her pelvic floor was NOT a disaster; she did NOT have pelvic floor dysfunction, vulvodynia, vulvar vestibulitis, or vulvar dysesthesia. Her doctor(s) got it all wrong. Abigail was normal. She had TMS, which is

---

\*The nocebo doesn't result from medical doctors only. It comes from many well-meaning health-practitioners such as, acupuncturists, masseuses, physical therapists, chiropractors and any other group that hands out guidance on problems with the physical body. The "helpful tips and advice" are common magnifiers of pain.

part of the human condition. Her doctor added his arcane terminology to her symptoms to try to define her problem, and in doing so, created a much worse situation by giving it life. The only thing he got right during the examination was when he said, "We really don't know why they (pain problems) occur." Had he known about Dr. Sarno's work he may have been able to help Abigail; instead, he contributed to her suffering.

Now what Abigail didn't know at the time, was that she was being prepared to help people. She had to first experience what they would be going through before she could be of help in the future. Experiencing chronic pain and fighting her way to good health again made her want to help others who were also struggling. At that time, there were very few people talking about pelvic pain issues as being TMS. So she wanted to give people hope by showing them that the various pelvic pain syndromes she had experienced were simply mindbody effects. She became a life coach with a focus on mindbody healing and began working with sufferers, showing them how the pressures and stresses they put on themselves out of the desire to be good, perfect, or even worthy of love are causing their pains.

Another contributor to the pain problems are the **testing triggers**, where the physician tests the sufferer in order to diagnose the problem, and the testing procedure itself triggers a new problem. This is seen quite a bit in urethral testing, where the sufferer's brain then latches onto the discomfort of the testing, and then can't let go of that new diversion, much like lifting something and hearing a popping sound in the spine.

Every day in doctor's offices, and across the Internet, people are being harmed by *myths*, *lies*, and *confusion*. Well-meaning institutions and kind individuals hand out harmful advice in the attempt "to help" (Refer to Appendix D). Pointing to the physical body as the cause of pain throws gasoline on a smoldering problem, codifying it into consciousness, generating victims, increasing tension, and empowering the deception. People are generally unaware of how powerful the mind is in health and healing, and so, they laugh at people who are aware.

But the sufferers must also believe and accept the error in order to host it. Once medically cleared for life-threatening issues, it's imperative to ignore everything you think you know about pain, and to get rid of all advice, gimmicks, and gadgets.

*If you are to do well, in getting rid of the (pain) problems you have now, you would do well to forget everything you've ever been told.*

John E. Sarno, MD[64]

## Not Another Pain in the Neck

In 2001, a whiplash study was reported in the "International Journal of Legal Medicine," entitled, "No Stress No Whiplash? Prevalence of Whiplash Symptoms Following Exposure to a Placebo Rear-end Collision."

Placebo studies are quite interesting; not only for what they supposedly reveal, but because they are so rare. This particular study, "No Stress No Whiplash,"[65] was set up using healthy volunteers who were recruited from a newspaper ad. The volunteers were subjected to a simulated rear-end collision through special effects. Their necks were stationary during the simulated collision, but their senses were subjected to the trauma of a virtual rear-end collision, using two standard European cars.

Immediately after the test, 18 percent of the participants reported neck symptoms; three days after, 20 percent reported neck symptoms; and four weeks later, 10 percent of the subjects complained of lingering neck pain. According to the study's designers, those subjects reporting neck pain, at all three stages of measurement, had "higher scores on the psychological scale of psychosomatic disorders ... significantly higher scores on emotional instability"... and higher scores on "whiplash-associated disorders." Repeatedly the evidence points toward personality and mental state as the greater indicators regarding suggestibility into pain, the need for pain as a diversion, and in its chronicity.

The conclusion drawn from the study, according to its designers, was that those volunteers who were under greater stress in their lives at "each post-trial measuring point" were the ones reporting longer effects of lingering symptoms. This also coincides with Dr. Sarno's lifework on TMS.

It also needs to be reemphasized that the lingering pain is not imagined, or faked—BUT it's also not from the body's structure. The volunteers' necks never moved during this experiment! Their senses **observed** a jarring event, and their bodies began to match and adapt to that **perception**. The only volunteers in this whiplash study whose biology began to match their perception of traumatic events were the ones under the greater psychic stress—who currently needed a diversion.

These are real physical mindbody effects—fueled by the power of expectation, driven by fear, and accelerated by financial reward. When the need for a diversion exists, those who are in need will latch onto whatever they can, using what their senses observe. Fear is the dis-ease that invites the pain to stay.

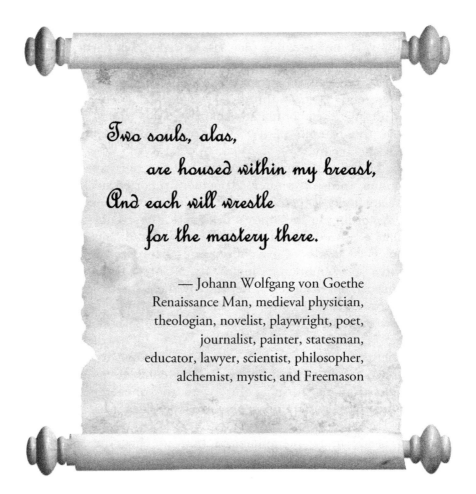

Two souls, alas,
     are housed within my breast,
And each will wrestle
     for the mastery there.

— Johann Wolfgang von Goethe
Renaissance Man, medieval physician,
theologian, novelist, playwright, poet,
journalist, painter, statesman,
educator, lawyer, scientist, philosopher,
alchemist, mystic, and Freemason

What's the most important part of your health?
What if I told you that caring for your body was
the least important part of your health? I'm a
physician, so if you had told me that five years
ago, I mean that would have been total
sacrilege, right? ... But what if I told you that
the medical profession had it all backwards? If
the body doesn't shape how we live our lives,
what if the body is actually a mirror of how we
live our lives ... Millions of people in this
country are ignoring the whispers of the body.
We're suffering from an epidemic that modern
medicine has no idea what to do with. People
suffering from this epidemic are fatigued,
they're anxious and depressed, they toss and
turn at night, they've lost their libido. They
suffer from a whole variety of aches and pains.

— Lissa Rankin, MD[67]

People will get an MRI (for back
pain), they'll have an abnormality,
that abnormality might have nothing
to do with their back pain, yet
because they have an abnormality in
the back and because they have back
pain, there's pressure on the
specialists to give treatment that
actually won't help them.

— John Mafi, MD, Beth Israel Deaconess
Medical Center[68]

... man creates his own illnesses

for a definite purpose, using the

outer world merely as an

instrument, finding there an

inexhaustible supply of material

which he can use for this purpose,

today a piece of orange peel,

tomorrow the spirochete of

syphilis, the day after, a draft of

cold air, or anything else that

will help him pile up his woes.

— Georg Groddeck, MD,
*Book of the It* (1923/1949)[69]

One of the most intriguing aspects of both hysterical and psychosomatic disorders is that they tend to spread through the population in epidemic fashion, almost as if they were bacteriological in nature, which they are not.

Edward Shorter, a medical historian, concluded from his study of the medical literature that the incidence of a psychogenic disorder grows to epidemic proportions when the disorder is in vogue. Strange as it may seem, people with an unconscious psychological need for symptoms tend to develop a disorder that is well known, like back pain, hay fever, or eczema. This is not a conscious decision. A second cause of such epidemics often results when a psychosomatic disorder is misread by the medical profession and is attributed to a structural abnormality.

— John E. Sarno, MD[70]

## Le Roy

In August of 2011, in Le Roy, NY, 14 students (13 girls and 1 boy) began experiencing tics, seizures, and vocal outbursts that mimicked Tourette's and/or PANDAS.* Initially, the town of Le Roy looked to the water source, as well as some form of contagious virus, as the culprit. However, an astute neurologist, Laszlo Mechtler, MD, from the Dent Neurologic Institute, quickly identified the problem as **conversion disorder**.† Conversion disorder occurs when a psychological stress manifests itself in a physical way, such as blindness, loss of speech, deafness, tics, paralysis, seizures, or pain.

Predictably, the families were offended—outraged at the conversion disorder diagnosis, and began demanding a biological answer to the physical problems, as do most sufferers with back pain. In the meantime, the Tourette-like symptoms were "infecting" more children, due to magnified media attention. The bigger the Le Roy story became on the local and national news, the more girls who became infected with similar symptoms. After Erin Brockovich was invited to town to test for chemical pollution, some of the girls began to cry that they were damaged for life by the chemicals that were in their head.

But there were no chemicals. The symptoms were psychological in nature. Each girl passed the disorder onto the next one, and the mind of each girl was fooled into thinking that the disorder began within her.

> *What the eyes see and the ears hear, the mind believes.*
> Harry Houdini

Le Roy was a classic case of meme transfer, amplified by mass hysteria. The town was so intensely obsessed with fear over the possibility of environmental pollution and infectious streptococcal bacteria as the culprit, that they missed the cause, which was a psychological need for a physical conversion. Fortunately for the children, the Dent Institute got it right. One child was diagnosed with Tourette's (the meme host child) and the other children fell prey to her symptoms. The afflicted children had unconsciously transmitted each other's tics and outbursts, and flinching—absorbing into themselves and then reflecting the original girl's symptoms. This is social contagion through **observational learning**. The most influential factors that increase the likelihood of imitation in observational learning are:

- When a situation is confusing;

---

*Pediatric Autoimmune Neuropsychiatric Disorders Associated with Streptococcal Infections.
†Conversion disorder was once known as *hysteria.*

- People are similar in age, sex, and interests;

- Lack of confidence.

The afflicted children of Le Roy had all these factors before them, and of course, the deeper personal need to express their problems through their bodies.

> *Illnesses hover constantly above us, their seed blown by the winds, but they do not set in the terrain unless the terrain is **ready** to receive them.*
>
> Claude Bernard, MD, father of physiology

## Reaction Formation

It was slowly revealed over time that the distressed Le Roy children had been under overwhelming psychic stress at home. And as with back pain—they unconsciously chose a form of expression that was observable, in vogue, and all around.

Back pain, as with conversion disorder, emanates from the sufferer's need to divert anxiety, and to be heard when they feel alone. Sufferers need to feel connected when they're frightened, and confused. They often pin their hopes to their doctors, anxiously anticipating that they will listen when no one else is paying attention. Their body is their only means of expression when they don't know how to verbally express their great angst. Suffering people need to be heard—connected—which is why talk therapy and journaling work so well in healing. But because no one is listening, and because of their inability to feel and express fear and anger, their problems are necessarily realized physically.[*]

> *He (Rosario Trifiletti, MD, pediatric neurologist, who set out to prove that the problem was **not psychological**, but rather bacterial) listened to our story, and right then he said, "This is definitely not conversion disorder," and that made me so happy, because finally someone was listening.*
>
> Lori Brownell, Le Roy, afflicted girl

Adding to the confusion in many mindbody disorders, and in cases such as Le Roy's, often exists an unconscious psychological defense mechanism called **reaction formation**. Defense mechanisms are in place to protect ego and to reduce anxiety. Reaction formation is a psychological defense whereby the ego attempts to avoid shame by pretending to adhere to the opposite impulse by distorting the unwanted

---

[*]Somaticizing is the inner-self, expressing itself, through the body—anxiety converted to physical symptoms.

and unconscious impulses into acceptable forms. In other words, sometimes people behave in an opposite manner to hide their true feelings; e.g., if someone hates someone, and may want to kill them, they may become overly nice to that person to hide the objectionable impulse of wanting to harm them. They disown their socially unacceptable impulse by casting it into their shadow. This is seen in Stockholm Syndrome and in abused children who run to the arms of the abuser. It's also seen in cases of reformed smokers and drinkers who go around extolling the sinful dangers of such acts—to cover their deep desire to drink and smoke, *to protect the ego from the id.*

> *A phobia is an example of a reaction formation. The person wants what he fears. He is not afraid of the object; he is afraid of the wish for the object. The reactive fear prevents the dreaded wish from being fulfilled.*
>
> Calvin S. Hall (1954/1999)[71]

In the Le Roy case, the girls' egos had them convinced that everything at home was peaceful and content, in order to protect them from their shadow. They were on TV proclaiming that everything at home was fine and dandy. But it was wishful thinking on their part … their descriptions of their lives were the way the girls wanted life to be. It was a quintessential reaction formation.

New York Times journalist Susan Dominus did a magnificent job in reporting on the underlying issues that the girls were experiencing. According to Dominus, one child's mother was suffering from chronic pain and cancer and had just had her 13th brain surgery shortly before her daughter accepted the Tourette meme and her symptoms began. There were "breakups with boyfriends," a father who "battled drug and alcohol addictions," leaving one daughter "emotionally abandoned, and physically abused."

Through reaction formation the girls had created a life of Pollyannaish perfection, in their minds. But there was high tension in their households that they were trying to cope through. Once the girls hit their emotional threshold, where they could no longer contain their fear, their brains were primed for an acceptable diversionary outlet to come along. The in-vogue story in town happened to be the Tourette's-like phenomenon on the local and national news—being talked about in every home in town.

> *Everyone had some sort of precipitant argument at school amongst friends, a breakup with a boyfriend, (for) a couple of the individuals it was just a life of a lot of hardship, and once we kinda opened Pandora's Box—if you will—things started to come out.*
>
> Jennifer McVige, MD, neurologist, Dent Institute[72]

## Similarities Between Le Roy and Back Pain

- The girls resisting an emotional cause for their problem were the ones still suffering, fishing for red herrings.

- The girls all either underestimated the stress they were under, or pretended it didn't exist.

- Those directly involved were insulted when they were told their physical problem was originating from a psychological process.

- They focused on the wrong measures to promote healing.

- Those accepting that the problem was psychological in nature were the ones healing.

- Those given a medical cure (antibiotics) began to experience a placebo response (healing response).

- This was reaction formation: they were not what they were pretending to be.

- They needed to be heard, to feel connected.

When a baby cries and someone comes to it, it is immediately conditioned to understand that crying brings someone when it needs and wants to feel connected. But what happens when it's no longer acceptable for superego to cry, beyond a certain age? The illnesses and pains can then unconsciously become substitutes for crying, as acceptable ways to pull those to us when we deeply need to feel safe, and loved.

> *Lori's (one of the girls afflicted) family is still resisting the idea of a psychological cause, and she continues to suffer from nonstop ticking*[72].

Back pain, much like conversion disorder, is a defense mechanism that can be observed. People do not inherit back pain; it's not genetic. The notion of back pain is transferred and absorbed through the current environment, whether it's at work, at home, or at play. The proof that back pain is not inherited is in the fact that sufferers heal even if their parents had the same type of pain. What they've actually inherited from their parents is worry.

> *I have observed, clinically, that back pain is "learned behavior." We learn from our parents, or others, that back pain (or other TMS symptoms), is a socially acceptable outlet, acting as a distraction, to keep us from thinking about things we don't want to think about.*
> Paul Gwozdz, MD, TMS physician, personal correspondence

Everyone is memed together in the turbulence of confusion. A meme is an unconscious unit of cultural replication, traveling from one brain to another; whether wanted or unwanted.

## Please Please Me ... *"C'mon C'mon ...."*

The phrase "to please" is important in understanding intermittent healing (placebo = *to please*). What the individual believes is going to help her, will help her. It pleases her, and so it eases her, because she deeply believes it is helping her, even if its only value is that it is acceptable to her. If she does not believe that something will help her, then it has little or no effect on her. This is readily seen in every placebo trial, and in every naysayer of truth. What a person does not believe, will not help.

Ted Kaptchuk, OMD, has been a pioneer in the study of placebos for decades. He has witnessed people get better or worse from "pretend" acupuncture, and from pills that sufferers thought were pain pills, but contained only cornstarch.

At the turn of the 20th century, the prolific healer Georg Groddeck, MD, had noted that he could have two patients with the same diagnosis, and prognosis, but one would die, and the other would live. The outcomes, he observed, depended on what the ill person deeply believed was going to happen. The human physiology will not only adapt to match the individual's perception of his situation, but to his will to heal, or even live. If he perceives that a new medical technique or popular and reputable surgeon is going to benefit, then it more often works—because of his awe-inspiring power of belief.

If you **believe** your back pain is caused by one leg being shorter than the other, then it is. If you **believe** your back pain will be healed because a great surgeon is operating on you, then the surgery may work for you. If you **believe** that realigning your body's posture will take your pain away, then it might. If you **believe** that holding a magnet will heal your body, then good for you. If you **believe** that the new pain cream is your cat's-meow then you've finally found a magic cure for your pain.

> *Truly I tell you, if anyone says to this mountain, 'go throw yourself into the sea,' and does not doubt in their heart but believes that what they say will happen, it will be done for them.*

Jesus, *Mark* 11: 23

But if you **don't believe** ... that therapy or injections, or even TMS will work, then they will not work. The great entrepreneur Henry Ford said, "Whether you think you can, or whether you think you can't, you're right." We are defined by our beliefs, for good or for bad.

*Take the time to challenge yourself (to heal) because you are that powerful. You are that strong. Never, ever doubt how truly powerful you are.*

Peter Zafirides, MD, TMS-practitioner,
President and Medical Director of
Central Ohio Behavioral Medicine

It's what you believe in your heart that truly matters, because what you believe germinates into the genesis of life-altering action: allowing for, or disabling, healing. The willpower of belief directs energy, which in turn affects matter since matter is a form of energy.

Our deeper beliefs are substantiated when we witness others around us healing, or not healing. They become our truths, **as far as we can currently see**. So, should we disregard all placebos? No. But it's important to note that the true reason(s) for certain effects is still lurking in the shadows. The confusion on back pain continues because each individual and each professional is certain that what he or she is doing is the correct way ... buried somewhere inside the mass confusion is truth.

The "sanction of the medical code" can harm you. This means that if you believe you are a helpless victim of the current methods of treating pain, then you need to abandon them. The passivity to submit yourself to the industry, and to the failed ways of treating back pain, results directly from your unsound obligation to your physician, and to a failed system. Accepting something means buying into it, and buying into it means maintaining partial ownership. If you aid in a process that harms you, then you are the owner of your own demise. The only way to permanently heal back pain is to fully understand what is occurring, and to reject what has already failed. Healing does not come from programs, methods, or "to do lists." It comes from knowledge, followed by a belief in that knowledge.

# 11

# Giant Mistakes

## The Blind Men and the Elephant

The temporary successes using the multidisciplinary approaches for treating back pain is reminiscent of the fable "The Blind Men and The Elephant." It's the age-old teaching story of six blind men who had heard of an elephant, but naturally had never seen one. The basic story has been relayed throughout ancient nations, in many forms. The premise is that each blind man wanted to know what elephants look like, in order to "satisfy his own mind." So each man touched the elephant on only one part of the elephant's body; they then compared notes on what the elephant looked like. Each described the elephant in a different manner, such as: looking like a pillar, a basket, spear, wall, tree, and fan. The differences in opinions were because each man had touched different aspects of the elephant—but only one aspect. Each had touched one aspect of Truth, and in knowing only a single part, each created a flawed universe based on partial conclusions. This is a **fallacy of composition**: *assuming something is true for the whole picture because it's true of parts of the picture.*

I chose this example for several reasons. One was because of its importance in illustrating **subjective experience**, as it relates to the nature of Truth. Each blind man, like many pain practitioners, came to the wrong conclusion because each had only experienced part of the picture. Not only was each man physically blind, but also blinded by his own narrow view of knowledge—feeling he had the truer truth. Many health practitioners fall into this trap when they enter into their specialty.

However, primarily I chose this example because of its ending. The men disagreed until it became hostile, and personal. People can't even agree on the meaning of the story. Some have claimed that it describes the nature of Truth; others have argued that it concerns the rise in conflict over disagreement; and yet others see a larger meaning, whereby a sighted man walks by and describes the entire elephant all at once, and the men suddenly become aware that they're blind. Personally, I agree with Rumi's analysis on the nature of the elephant story: "If each had a candle, and they went in together, the differences would all disappear."

## Living Is Easy With Eyes Closed –
### *"Strawberry Fields Forever"*

The metaphor of "blind men" holds true for treating back pain, and pain in general. Many pain brokers have different vested interests in seeing his or her own interpretation accepted, and in discounting that Dr. Sarno's is not. The elephant in the room is the medical industry: big, powerful, lumbering, out of control, with everyone jumping on for a ride. The blind men represent both the sufferers and practitioners desperately grasping in the dark to satisfy their own mind. Dr. Sarno represents the man walking by and describing the entire picture—and suddenly everyone realizes they're blind.

If only people would get together, the problem could disappear. But that will never happen. Where there is vested self-interest, and ego, there will never be a mutual goal. People with healthy eyes look directly at TMS and walk away. They can't dispute it, so they turn a blind eye. Dr. Sarno had hoped that his colleagues would challenge his findings at some point, so that he could show them proof of his successes. But it never happened.

The *good doctor* saw the entire elephant, from above, and from below, and from inside out. Perhaps it takes a 50-year career to paint, and to frame, and to display such a comprehensive picture. Or maybe it just takes a physician who is willing to sit and listen to his patients. Thanks to Dr. Sarno, the message on how to heal back pain is powerful, and strong, and moving forward one giant step at a time.

# 12

# Healing Back Pain

## General Rules of Thumb

There are varying TMS approaches that can be used to heal back pain, and have been described in the many books available on TMS. The approach is not as important as recognizing that you have TMS, and not some incurable physical problem—as your doctor, masseuse, physical therapist, or neighbor might have told you. A simple and direct approach that I recommend is as follows:

- **First:** Get a physical exam. Protect your life.

- **Second:** If you're not dying or in danger, reject the diagnosis of a defective spine.

- **Third:** Accept the TMS diagnosis; i.e., your pain is not from the structure of your spine, it is originating from your autonomic nervous system, ANS.

- **Fourth:** Stop ALL forms of treatment to "heal" your back. There's nothing that needs healed.

  Then:

- **Avoid all tips and tricks:** from well-meaning websites, books, friends, and loved ones.

- **Start to gather TMS information:** it's everywhere now.

- **Live your life as though you were healed:** do everything you want to do.

- **Try to sense how you feel:** TMS back pain stems from not being aware of how you feel, at any point. Try to sense these emotions you've been blocking/repressing. Note them, but don't judge them or to try to react to them. Become aware of their existence.

- **Begin to connect your pain to your emotions:** feel your pain as anger/rage and fear and frustration, or sorrow. Reverse your perception: it's not a nerve-pinching sensation; it's actually a sucking/pulling sensation from a lack of oxygen.

- **Use Guided Imagery:** your biology adapts to align with your perception of your environment, as in the Le Roy case. So when you view your spine as being broken, flawed, deteriorating, and unfixable, then that's what you adapt to become. See your back as healthy and strong, which it is!

- **Breathe:** breathing is important. I recommend doing it many times every day. But beyond doing it to survive—begin relaxation techniques such as **conscious breathing** from the belly. Conscious breathing eases over-stimulation of the autonomic nervous system and lowers tension, allowing rebalancing to occur. Breathing is the doorway to the autonomic nervous system, where TMS emanates. The brain associates belly breathing with relaxation, and chest breathing with anxiety.

- **Look at your relationships:** TMS tension comes from conflict, and almost all conflict comes from within the family unit. Who is it that you're angry toward? Who have you been trying to pull to you, or push away? Many sufferers have reported that they healed once they forgave someone, or fell in love. Who has recently died, or divorced? Who is sick or missing? Who are you not talking to right now? Who are you taking care of right now? What do you feel guilty about, ashamed of, or sorry for? What is your biggest fear?

- **Use Self-talk:** affirmations have been a great source of healing because they reverse inaccurate thinking. Since TMS starts with negative self-blame and self-talk, it's useful to do the opposite. Pouring "accurate information" into your deeper brain forces it to give up its strategy of self-punishment and deceit. "I deserve love" is a great affirmation to keep going, but "I forgive" is the best way to start. When we hold resentment toward someone we chain ourselves to that person for life; we become their slave. When we truly forgive them we free ourselves, forever. As author of self-inquiry Byron Katie wrote, "Would you rather be right, or free?"

- **Stop thinking about what your body is doing:** don't grade your body every day. When you begin to go somewhere or do something, don't look at how your back is doing, or how your back will be. It's okay! Just go do it.

- **Let go of attachments:** objects do not bring happiness, relationships do. Let go of material attachments, as well as emotional attachments, such as resentment, frustration, hate, and sadness.

- **Stop physical therapy altogether:** stop trying to strengthen your core, stop trying to stretch for pain relief, stop trying to align your spine, stop trying to do anything for your body to relieve pain. Stop acupuncture, spinal adjustments, core stretching, strengthening ... everything. Stop trying to heal; you're prolonging your suffering. Physical therapy can make you worse.

- **Laugh more:** laughter creates the experience of anti-pain, such as joy, enabling the ability to free yourself from the shackles of guilt, and shame. Laughter releases dopamine (the reward hormone)—a neurotransmitter responsible for the feeling of pleasure that mitigates pain. The late Norman Cousins healed himself from crippling ankylosing spondylitis, a painful chronic inflammatory disease, using laughter as a primary tool. From his book *Anatomy of an Illness*, "I made the joyous discovery that ten minutes of genuine belly laughter had an anesthetic effect and would give me at least two hours of pain-free sleep[73]."

- **Stop talking about pain:** stop thinking about your body, stop peeking at its progress, stop telling people about your symptoms, stay away from pain groups that talk about pain. They reinforce the problems in the mind.

- **Journal:** people have reported that self-writing helped to dramatically ease their pain. The reason is clear: writing is expressing, and pain is the deeper-self attempting to express itself.

- **Talk therapy:** if your pain becomes relentless, or continues to move around, it's a good time to seek counseling or a respected spiritual leader. Let it out by talking (aka, chimney sweeping).

- **Learn how to say "no" to people:** their opinion doesn't matter in your life; learn how to say no to some people, at certain times.

- **Alter your perceptions:** your body is not failing, it's reacting to what you aren't aware of. Turn your current perception of stress into opportunity.

- **Become more physical:** when you have enough confidence that you have TMS, begin to do anything you want to do, without fear of hurting yourself. Dr. Sarno stated that this was **the most important thing one can do**.

The concept is to **never try to heal**—don't fight pain*; rather, remove all the barriers within you that you have placed to prevent healing. The information in this book is true, and it works virtually every time. If you refuse to believe it, the questions then become, "Why do you need your pain? Why are you protecting it?" The cell door, to the prison that you alone have constructed, is wide open. All you need to do is walk out and begin to enjoy your freedom.

---

*This isn't the same as becoming physically aggressive again. Physical exertion is necessary and should begin as soon as the sufferer is confident in the TMS diagnosis. "By not fighting it" I mean don't battle against yourself and against all the reasons for the pain, and never purposefully go out and attack the pain. Never do that! Attacking pain is falling right back into the brain's strategy. You can fight to become active again, and fight for hope again, but never fight for pain reduction. Become physical to free yourself, and for good health and the feeling of wellness.

Sometimes sufferers, after many years and decades in pain, heal quickly with this newfound knowledge, but this is rare. The normal path to healing is to dig deeper into the thinking and emotional factors and to allow for slow healing, as you integrate the new paradigm. If you want to know more, there is TMS information everywhere out there that can put you in a state that allows your mind to release your pain. There's also the TMSWiki.org, and of course, Dr. Sarno's great books.

## Complaining and Criticizing: *"Light on Application!"*

A few people will read this book, *Back Pain: Permanent Healing*, and say, "Hey ... that guy talked a lot about the controversy over back pain but very little about what to do about it—that book sucked!" But this is not a "how to" book, it's a "why" book. Understanding the whys leads to *permanent* healing. The how-to books along with all the "methods, gadgets, and programs" have made back pain the number one global disability in the world. However, "not enough practical information on what to do" is a common criticism for the topic of TMS literature. Healing is not a matter of saying, "Do X, Y, and Z," and you will heal. It doesn't work that way. There's no panacea beyond consciousness. People often buy self-healing books hoping that this new one will have the magic formula. They scour through the pages looking for actions to take. But there are no miraculous words, or actions beyond self-knowledge. The better books can only enlighten with information, they can't provide healing. The author tries to phrase the wording so that it profoundly connects with the reader in a new and clearer way. And so repeated reading of the correct information is the answer, not more information.

 The searching for answers that are already here is a defense against healing.

Each sufferer must recognize within themselves that they're not who they're pretending to be, that they are pulled out of balance, that they're killing themselves with self-imposed demands, that they're lonely and disconnected, that their body is not flawed, and that their pain is from unfelt emotions. They then need to change their lives by changing their perception of themselves. Nothing can do that for them, but them.

"Healing" takes emotional insight, belief, realization, gathering of small truths, reflection, failing, tenacity, courage, change, and the piecing together of the personal psyche. So of course a few will say this book sucks, but—there's a reason for that (not the sucking part ... the not talking very much about "how to heal" part). Here's why:

First, this book is an argumentative outline of what's working and what isn't, in the effort to shed more light, and to help suffering people understand deeper why they haven't been successful in their healing. Understanding the argument itself is part of the healing process, regarding the covert methods of the brain: ego shielding truth, hiding shame, physical diversions, guilt, excuses, procrastinating, and defense mechanisms, among many other self-deceptions.

Second, there is no one way to heal, no cookie-cutter method that can be written down to be followed step by step. If that were the case the method shouldn't work! If it did there also would be no need for doctors or therapists. The "grinding through on your own" is the individuating process of healing. If you were to follow me, or anyone else, you'd be falling right into the trap of social contagion that got you here. Healing varies from person to person, depending on how that person's ego hides shame and guilt. It's a personal and sometimes dark journey that each person must traverse on his own. But it sometimes helps to have a streetlight along the way, to see a direction. So on occasion, a structured step-by-step process can be a generic guide. But in my opinion, the de-structuring of life begins the permanent healing because it's the worry of responsibility, and of always trying to do things right that generates much of the tension.

Another reason it's not important to spell out healing is that the emperor is still naked. You've either made an immediate connection with what I've written here, or you haven't. But there are many who continue to complain that the healing book(s) don't talk enough about "what to do!?"* These are revealing statements on where the individual is in understanding, and in how far away they are from healing.

Hopefully, your pain won't have to get much worse before you're ready to listen, as was my case. Those who can see this light will immediately go find all the TMS information they can, and slowly begin letting go. If they don't believe this message, then why waste their time by including more tedious betawave-generating detail in a book? Furthermore, the best I can do for anyone who wants to heal from back pain is to show them TMS ... and then explain why it's so controversial. In the time skeptics devote to disputing this proven message, they could have already begun healing. But pain, like illness, is a very personal thing: not only in the need for the sensation of pain, but also in the rejection of the information that can help.

The need to be spoon-fed answers has two aspects:

---

*There are plenty of things "to do" mentally. This refers to the "act of healing," or trying to heal an already healthy body. "What to do" is a learning process, not a body-healing process. Knowing the difference is important in healing.

- The person in severe pain has less patience for learning, and desires a quick out, which is quite understandable. Pain certainly destroys patience.

- They're resisting healing. Statements such as, "It was light on application" are indicative of the continuing need for a diversion. The use of the "not enough" straw man is to put off the changes necessary to heal.

*The Great Pain Deception* took 10 years to write and publish. It is 377 pages, with 330 citations, over 200 pages of information on psychology and the human mind; it includes philosophy, real-life examples of healing, and studies described in chapters such as, "What You Need to Understand to Heal." Some readers have reported needing two or three months to read through and to digest because it's packed with choco-licious information on healing. TMS expert Dr. Paul Gwozdz stated, "I consider *The Great Pain Deception* to be the definitive encyclopedia of TMS." And yet, a couple people have commented, "I wish it would have told me more about what to do." These poor folks can't see the forest because of all the trees in their way. But they will see it all come together when they are **ready**.

A large portion of the healing process is to stop following other people's leads, to take **your own life** back, to find **your** path, to stop relying on **their** opinions. Go ... find **your** own way.

## Weaning off the Spoon: Healing Thyself

*Healing Back Pain* was the only TMS book needed for me to let go of 30 years of pain. I found a way to heal from its information. However, others have written to me saying, "I know Dr. Sarno is right, but he left me somewhat hanging on what to do." I never felt that way, I saw his core message immediately ... so I went out to make the changes in my life necessary to stop the punishing cycle. I wanted to heal; but more important, after so much suffering, I was **finally ready** to allow the truth. The concept of needing to be fed sordid details is a larger narrative in the entire **trouble healers** topic.

People will sometimes contact me to ask for someone's name who has healed from back pain, shoulder, foot, knee pain, or fibromyalgia, etc., who they can talk to, as more proof. But I try to explain that the other person can't do it for them. Ordinarily, when I give them a name, they unfailingly want another, and then another.* The same is true for healing timeframes. The majority of people ask, "How long did it take for that person to heal from their '___' pain?" But how long it took someone else is irrelevant, their healing time has nothing to do with your healing. It's like asking how long it took for the other person to become happy, and then trying to become happy inside their timeframe. The same light shines on the diamond and the coal, but only the diamond reflects the light within because it is **ready** to shine.

It's quite understandable to be curious as to how others have fared though—life is all about **connection**. We feel better if someone else has gone through it and recovered. Their example lowers our fear factor and gives us a template to follow. Their model is the light that guides us out of our own darkness. I wholly recognize how powerful examples are, as some helped me heal; but a couple examples are enough. Demanding superfluous information is procrastinating on the hard work. You either see it, or you don't. The perverted emperor will just not cover himself up. This is often an unconscious defense mechanism by the brain called **intellectualization**.† But be of great cheer, you *can* heal; and you *will* heal, if you turn around and begin to see how you got here.

## From Coal to Diamond

Within these pages is what I've learned about what works, and what I have seen that stagnates healing. I wrote this book to help people, to pull the light from them that already exists within them. Some will learn, and some won't, but I am obligated to try to help. *To whom much is given....*

> *These structural abnormalities are real, and they are there, but they are not the cause of the pain. This is an enormous misconception in medicine ... there is no evidence in the medical literature that this is so (that herniated discs cause pain).*
>
> John E. Sarno, MD[74]

I either had some readers, or lost them, in the first sentence of this book when I wrote: "Back pain rarely, if ever, comes from herniated discs or spinal narrowing, and it certainly never comes from spinal or core weakness, slipped discs, or spinal misalignment." A few folks will

---

*This form of resistance is also seen when a sufferer gets the TMS diagnosis from a TMS physician, and then wants to find another TMS physician to confirm the first diagnosis, and then another, etc.

†Intellectualization reduces anxiety by remaining distant from the reality of the situation. Focusing on intellectual aspects only (learning, reading), in a cold clinical manner helps avoid the unacceptable emotions.

have read on to the end, to obtain more ammunition to refute what's already working.

> **John Stossel:** *So week after week these people who've seen a dozen doctors to no avail, come to you, and they get better?*
>
> **Dr. Sarno:** *Yes ... virtually all of them.*
>
> ABC 20/20[75]

Some readers may just want a few more details on what to do, and of what not to do. That's good! You've already begun reversing your pain if you're curious. When billionaire Warren Buffet was asked about how much money he was going to leave his children when he died, he said, "I'm going to leave them enough so that they can do anything they want, but not so much that they don't have to do anything at all." Once you accept that your pain is coming from unfelt emotions, you have to start getting down to work, with just enough help to keep you standing; but not so much help that you don't have to use your own legs.

## Helping People Heal

> *The most helpful tip for me (from Steve) was 'do nothing to heal my (back) pain.' It exploded through my body and mind. (Then) one August day there was a breakthrough for me, it happened, the pain stopped. It was a miracle to me.*
>
> Ales Kezman, Slovenia
> former back pain sufferer[76]

From my experience, it's sometimes more beneficial to tell people what NOT to do, than what to do.

- Don't try to heal.

- Don't complicate healing. People will sometimes meet me with pencil and paper in hand, ready to create a list of daily, minute-by-minute activities "to do." For example, at 11:03 AM laugh, at 11:07 AM look out the window, at 11:19 AM journal for 30 minutes, etc. Transformation comes from the opposite of that type of structured thinking. They more often need to un-structure their lives, impose fewer self-demands, reduce the pressure to be perfect and to heal perfectly. They're in pain because they want too much control, demand too much of themselves, and hold onto too many attachments. Keep healing simple, keep life simple. Live, laugh, and love. Some people are off enjoying life while others are analyzing it.

- Stop the cycle of thinking that creates the pain: stop planning, thinking about body, about what can go wrong, what others have, and how long others take to heal.

- You are not who you are pretending to be, so don't be "the you" that you're trying to be for everyone else. Your persona was formed by the outside world. Be the "you" who isn't living for them. Don't adjust to the demands of everyone else; they're trying to solve their own problems. The idea is to not be someone who lives a false-self in order to gain love from others, but to find ways to give more love to other people.

The faster healers don't want more proof. Some have healed while I was talking to them, others while grinding through the books. They don't need another example. To paraphrase the fastest healers as a group, from their collective emails and phone calls: "Oh my god Steve ... oh my god!! Dr. Sarno is soooo right, I just know this is me, I just know I have TMS, thank you so much, why doesn't everyone know about this? And why is the emperor standing over there naked?"

Those people go on to heal ... very nicely. The rest heal, too, but they need more insight, more confidence, more support, and more time. They move with greater caution. The rate of healing depends on the degrees of cynicism, fear, and belief. But the most important factor is **the need** for the pain. If you need your pain to hide your fear and rage,* your shame, your life, and your Self, then you may **resist healing**. The ones resisting healing the most are the ones who:

- Keep saying, "But my doctor told me I have ....";
- Keep refusing to ever get off their meds;
- Keep seeking other methods/techniques beyond TMS;
- Keep reading about TMS;†
- Keep talking about their body;
- Keep wanting free help only;‡
- Keep demanding more examples;
- Keep rolling their eyes;
- Keep complaining, "But, there's no science behind this."

TMS is the cause of almost all back pain in the world. And the TMS philosophy of healing is a clinically proven concept. In reality, the process works. Those demanding more science behind it are asking for theoretical proof. They don't care that it's working for the TMS physicians, therapists, coaches, counselors, and psychologists. They

---

*I'll put this footnote here as a reminder. People much too often say, "But I don't feel any rage!" Again, it's **unconscious**, you can't feel it. If you felt it, you would have no pain. The pain is the rage.
†They keep reading even after they understand it well.
‡Unless they truly can't afford help; which is a wholly different scenario.

don't care that every day people are healing around the world with the news that Dr. Sarno shared. They demand that it be theoretically proven in an experimental laboratory situation. To them, the fact that it works in reality means nothing. This is resistance.

This is not to say that anyone who needs a bit more information will never heal. The cynical brain just moves with greater caution in some folks. One cautionary shield is to argue over what Dr. Sarno proved to be right, by commenting, "I don't agree with Dr. Sarno because of this ...." Some feel that they know more about Dr. Sarno's work than he does. These people sometimes heal, too, but only in the manner in which they have decided will work, by finding a facet that *pleases them.* It's a personal journey of enlightenment, discovered on the dark and lonely road to within. Resistance represents the potholes in the entire process. The road is much bumpier for those who take the side roads to their own destination. Facing the Self can be painful, but there are lessons to be learned no matter which road we travel because there is no wrong road. The road you travel was the one you needed to take at that time.

*There is no coming to consciousness without pain*[77]. *People will do anything, no matter how absurd, in order to avoid facing their own Soul*[78]. *One does not become enlightened by imagining figures of light, but by making the darkness conscious*[79].

CG Jung, MD

## Third Eye Open

The acceptance of Truth/Self can be difficult, but is worth every effort. People end up happier, more balanced, more grounded, and more at peace with themselves and with others around them. They resist less within, and therefore without. They begin to observe life from the other side as they suddenly see themselves in everyone else. They're more attuned, in tune, and aware—ready to adapt to the next challenge that comes their way. Instead of repressing and resisting, they express themselves, and flow into the situation. They speak up when they feel they've been wronged but they still respect others' opinions. They become more actively engaged in daily life: helping, listening, laughing, and loving. They begin to see the elegant design in everything, and how we are all tied together. They also see TMS in everyone around them.

If you can't change, you can't heal. Consciousness is not a matter of left or right, up or down, right or wrong. It's the result of the understanding of the differences among these aspects.

## How Do I Forgive?

On occasion, people will ask me how they can forgive someone, or how to stop being angry at someone. These are experiential perceptions that one person cannot relay to another person. One person can't teach another how to let go of anger, or how to forgive. Forgiveness is a personal sensation of justice, encouraged by ego. True healing comes not from figuring these quandaries out, but in more fully understanding why you react the way that you do.

When there is TMS back pain there is hidden tension from unexpressed anger, disguised by ego. Tension comes from separation. The separation creates fear, resulting in the feelings of anger, resentment, and sorrow. Tension increases when pretending to care, while simultaneously not caring. Pretending to be someone, but not being that person at all.

The mother of anger is fear, sired by low self-esteem. Healing is incumbent upon the reversal of self-image—from no value, to great value. You won't be anxious when you're no longer angry. You won't be angry, when you no longer fear. You'll no longer fear when you no longer feel alone. You'll no longer feel alone when you find Truth.

## Whine Not

Why not try TMS healing? Why complain about it? It's free, it's safe, and it's proven. Nothing is certain when you begin to mess with the human body to fix it. I was thrilled when I saw Dr. Sarno offering a way to heal back pain without surgery or injections, because my ex-wife was permanently paralyzed from the waist down from a spinal injection. She was made a paraplegic for life from a relatively routine and minor procedure (which is an example of how fairly routine procedures carry no guarantees). The tragedy is that many other tragedies could have been avoided with TMS knowledge. But we live and learn. If we live but never learn we become targets of what we haven't learned, the very arrows we ourselves have fired.

## Methylprednisolone

In 2012, an outbreak of fungal meningitis occurred when several contaminated lots of Methylprednisolone killed 64 people and left over 750 ill, many with a strongly resistant infection.

Methylprednisolone is an epidural steroid injection, ESI, used to treat back pain. The contaminated injections were traced back to a company called the New England Compounding Center. A lengthy investigation showed that the company had used expired ingredients, failed to follow standards for cleanliness, and had violated its state license on how it prepared and shipped the drug. As a result of the willful negligence, fourteen people faced charges ranging from racketeering to fraud, and interstate sale of adulterated drugs.

It's truly a misfortune all around, especially when there's no evidence that steroid injections reduce back pain. None. But it doesn't stop doctors from prescribing them, just like with discectomies. Boston University law professor, Kevin Outterson commented on the Methylprednisolone tragedy in The New England Journal of Medicine stating:

> *But it's important to note that many patients received these sterile injections for back and joint pain, a procedure that lacks high-quality evidence of efficacy. These problems cannot be laid entirely at the feet of compounders when clinicians persist in clinical practices despite weak evidence of efficacy*[80].

Doctors prescribe steroid injections with great hope. But there's no evidence that they do anything, which is what Dr. Sarno had been stating all along. They may have had a patient or two that had a nice placebo response, or they may just be prescribing ESIs because everyone else is. Epidural steroid injections are part of the failed multidisciplinary and medical industry approaches to dealing with back pain.

It's impossible to ever know—but if we can reasonably extrapolate what we currently know about TMS onto this tragic situation, it's highly probable that most of those poor folks who received the Methylprednisolone never had to die. They never needed the injections. We'll never know for certain; the needle and the damage are done.

## The End Is Simply the Beginning

Healing from back pain may come from any number of insights, personal revelations, and "ah-ha" moments. The healing tool is the **knowledge** of what is truly going on, followed by the application of **belief**. All the knowledge in the world won't help if you don't believe it. Healing requires seeing and accepting a side of yourself that you have disowned. Once you've accepted that your spine is okay, healing is on its way.

I'll offer a final word of advice to those who want to try TMS healing. The idea is not to become a better person, or greater ... but rather to un-become everything you are not. People try to heal by changing everything around them, or their environment; but all healing comes from unblocking the truth within. The fact that they're suffering means they're not being true to themselves, and are ignoring their own needs.

When they begin to move beyond the pretense of what they're pretending to be, they become happier. Once they're happier, their suffering ends—and it begins with Knowledge of Truth.

Can anyone disagree that the happiest people are the ones being truer to their nature? When we're acting in accordance with our nature, as people of enlightenment, we have more confidence, more energy, and we add value to the world. In many surveys that ask about "attractiveness," both men and women answer that the most attractive trait in the opposite sex is **confidence**. Confident people are less conflicted, more relaxed, their paths straighter and narrower. Fear no longer pushes them to act; they are pulled along by light. We don't need more information to become who we are, only to listen to our heart. An important step in healing is in melting the frozen Self. If you're suffering, then you're not doing what you want, saying what you want, or acting like you want. You're placing too much pressure on yourself to please, and never fail.

## Healing Material

The world is saturated with healing information. The TMS books should be first on the list. After that, there is other material that can certainly help—offshoots of TMS—that may be of some value, depending on what the sufferer needs to hear in order to connect, and to release doubt. There's always something that can help based on what the specific need is. If the desire to heal is there, the information already exists. *Seek, and ye shall find ...* and know that what you seek already exists and is also seeking you. No matter what, someone still needs to get the emperor a robe, a towel, boxers, anything?!

## What Is Real Healing?

Healing begins when you realize at the deepest level that there's nothing physically wrong with your body's structure—when you can do anything you want to do with very little or no pain, AND ... when you no longer fear your pain. If these criteria are met, you are healed. You're "almost healed" when you no longer care "when" healing occurs. You're well on your way at that point. If your pain is gone but you are still afraid of doing certain activities, then you are not quite healed in its truest sense. You may feel better, which is good, but your brain is still using fear in you. Sometimes it only takes a small change in understanding, and sometimes it takes a life transformation. Between the two ends of the spectrum is a life well lived.

## The Tree Is Known by Its Fruit

> *To avoid criticism, say nothing, be nothing, do nothing.*
>                                                    Aristotle

In many ways, the health practitioners, whose purpose is to teach and strengthen us, have instead weakened us—by convincing us that we are weak, frail and susceptible, in need of constant repair. Through the years, many who are deemed scholarly and qualified have passed down poor information under the social armor of being "credentialed." People often become irate at their health practitioners once they discover TMS. They realize they were made to jump through many painful hoops, needlessly. But I often find myself in the ironic position of defending those in healthcare because I receive communication from practitioners who discover TMS, see its truth, and then quickly adjust their practices accordingly. These insightful ones include medical doctors, chiropractors, and acupuncturists, among others. There are good people all around who truly care.

## Cast Not Your Line Outward

Criticizing/judging of others is a means of control. Criticizing is more often **projecting**, which is a strategy by ego to make the judger feel better about himself. He points to the problem in you, so that he doesn't have to look at the same problem in himself. This is vital to understand in healing back pain because rejection is at the core of the eternal longing to be connected. However, as Jung stated, "Everything that irritates us about others can lead us to a better understanding of ourselves." So there are lessons to be learned all around.

Be aware of **reactivity**[*] while on the healing journey. Lessen your internal resistance, and allow your pain to fade. Soften your anger at doctors, and all of those with whom you disagree. The fight with others is a reflection of the fight within you. Learn to love yourself, or you can never deeply love others. Hate yourself and you will find problems in everyone around you.

Knowledge is information, experience is wisdom.

---

[*]**Reactivity** is reacting "automatically" the same way every time, meaning that our shadow is in control of us. Two signs of reactivity are: 1) scripting, responding the same way every time; and 2) overreacting, through a disproportionate response. We need to relate to our shadow's reactions and not to pretend they aren't happening. The goal is to realize when you are engaging in reactivity.

A couple months after I published my first book, people began healing with the information in it. When the very first person contacted me to say they had healed, it was a huge relief: "Whew ... it worked!!" Someone was listening. Someone was **ready** to heal. It was such a special moment, such a surreal feeling. However, later, in the middle of the first few hundred healing emails one disbeliever wrote this to me: "Back pain can come from any source and it has nothing to do with one's unconscious, or personality! I can attest to the fact that herniated discs and sciatica DO cause pain, and so will millions of others!" The emailer then went on to chastise me about selling snake oil to desperate people, and that he would be "keeping an eye on me!" Besides trying to figure out what snake oil is, I acknowledged that I had been forewarned. The email ended by telling me that he had "five college degrees, one of which is in psychology!"—and that, "My father was a doctor!" My first thought while reading that email was of the Hindu proverb, *"The birth of ego is the death of wisdom."*

This multi-degreed individual is a treasure of psychological case studies. But most important, he needed his opinion made known. He was 40 years behind in his understanding of back pain, but I under-stood his desperate need to be heard, and to feel relevant. At some point in his life he felt he was not being heard, his opinion not valued. So he went out and obtained five degrees so that he would have a soapbox from which he could shout—tossing around accomplishments as proof of knowledge, and carrying credentials as self-worth. I have college degrees myself, but none of them helped me with understanding The Mindbody Syndrome, or in relieving my suffering. This skeptic had been drawn into Dr. Karen Horney's third method[81] for coping, which Karen called: "unassailability."

When a child doesn't get enough attention from parents, Dr. Horney observed that the child would choose one of three classifications for survival:

- **Compliance**—going along, not making waves, a yes-person;

- **Aggression**—going against, making "anti"-waves, a no-person;

- **Unassailability**—going out and accomplishing; achieving much, getting many degrees, gathering awards, and trophies, so that they can never be rejected, or challenged in their positions. They feel that having accomplishments makes them wiser. But only experience makes us wiser, and suffering is the accelerator of that experience. The darkness is burned by the light; the light cannot be extinguished by darkness. Ignorance is darkness, and Truth is Light. The choice to spread light, or to live in darkness, determines the life that will be lived, or not lived.

The Sufi-poet wrote that there are three ways to know fire. One way is to hear about the fire, the other is to see the fire, and the third is to be burned by the fire. Experience is the supreme teacher. Listen to those who have been burned by suffering, and have healed; they're the ones who understand at the level of wisdom, through their scars of experience. Knowledge is information, it can be passed along to others in the healing process, but experience is wisdom; it cannot be given to anyone else, and comes only from within. Wisdom is the destruction of ego and is stored in consciousness; it cannot be obtained through education which is only a memory. When thinking dissolves into awareness you will come to your own truth, alone in stillness, and suffering ends.

## Two Pillars of Enlightenment

The works that most influenced my understanding, and aided in my being able to piece together my healing, were from two men: John Sarno and Clancy McKenzie. Dr. McKenzie discovered a Two-Trauma Mechanism identifying the relationship between early trauma (perceived emotional abandonment) and the later development of emotional disorders that lead to health disorders. Indeed, Dr. McKenzie's work supports Dr. Sarno's, and vice versa, although I'm sure neither man ever knew the other.* They both stood firm in the face of critics and cynics, spreading light with their groundbreaking discoveries, and unbending courage. Yet they were rejected by many of their professional peers.

Both changed the world by observing something that repeatedly held true, and both were met with the greatest resistance from the "educated ones." Both men stated that the laymen understood their concepts fairly easily. I recall statements that each made, that perhaps represented their culmination of frustration.

> **From Dr. Sarno:** *I have demonstrated conclusively that a truly physical-pathological process is the result of emotional phenomena, and can be halted by a mental one. That is, first of all, rank heresy, and secondly, beyond the comprehension of most physicians ... paradoxically, thoughtful laymen are much more able to accept such an idea because they are not burdened with a medical education and all the philosophical biases that go along with it.*

---

*Dr. Sarno clinically proved that **unconscious anger**, "to the point of rage," caused most of our health problems. The anger and rage are social reactions to our **fear**. Dr. McKenzie's work shows where the majority of our fear-induced-rage comes from: **separation trauma**. The fear of being alone, separate, isolated: the perception of emotional abandonment causes the anger behind TMS.

**From Dr. McKenzie:** *Too often persons do not trust their own minds to evaluate simple things; and they await the opinions of others before casting their lot. This holds true even for professionals in high places.*

## Pain Is Stored in the Shadow

The brilliant Swiss psychiatrist, Carl Jung said, "The **shadow** is that thing we have no wish to be." It is our undeveloped self ... self-serving, needy, and frightened. But our shadow is also our inner gold—if we know how to dig for it, how to use it. We do everything we can to overcome its shame and shortcomings. Indeed, many of our current strengths today were once our greatest weaknesses that we were shamed into overcoming. Our darkness helps to make us whole, if we choose light first, but also accept that we possess both light and dark.

*This earth is nothing but movies to me. Just like the beam of a motion picture. So is everything made of shadows and light. That's what we are, light and shadows of the Lord, nothing else than that. There's one purpose: To get to the beam. We are light and shadows of the Lord, that's all.*

Paramahansa Yogananda,
"Awake: The Life of Yogananda"

Beware of people wielding accomplishments and degrees as weapons. Many of them are the ones who got us into this mess of pain epidemics. They may have obtained their positon to hide their own weaknesses. Or they may just be brilliant messengers of light. Each person is unique, and driven by personal motivations. But certainly, the true person of science will keep an open mind, and the person of self-interest will close his, and try to close the minds of others. The difference is in the thirst for Truth (desire to get back to the beam). One becomes qualified in order to boast, to avoid rejection, and to make Mom proud—the other wants to make a difference. John Sarno and Clancy McKenzie made a world of difference. I'm sure their moms would be proud.

*I don't have a college degree, and my father didn't have a college degree. So when my son Zachary graduated from college, I said, My boy's got learnin!*
Robin Williams, gone but not forgotten

Whether you're a layman or professional, when you see something that's working, that is helping people recover from great suffering, the right thing would be to jump in and help, not to figure out ways to destroy it. TMS is coming; it can't be stopped.

I have ruminated on what Dr. Sarno taught us with his keen insight and bravery. Every time I think I have the answer, the answer changes.

But I believe that ultimately we will come to know that he **empowered us** to heal ourselves, by showing us that we are much stronger than we've been led to believe. He also unveiled to us who we really are, and what we truly aren't. By knowing we are okay, the guided image of ourselves has changed from "dis"-abled, to abled. The new image then becomes our future, which is a very bright future.

This book is about a healing message, a conversational argument on back pain. But it also describes almost all of our other common ailments. I explored the reasons that people are so confused, as well as the mythology that has grown from the aspiration for profit, and relevancy. I ended with some of the lies of rejection that are trying to obfuscate and disrupt this groundbreaking news. We can also look back on the past 100 years and see that many of the surgeries on knees, shoulders, hands, feet, and backs were unnecessary procedures. But the many placebo outcomes were enough for the industry and the populace to go along with the elusory results. The newer placebo trials are proving this to be true.

As I began, I will end. Back pain is the #1 cause of job disability in the entire world, but it does not have to be. Healing often only requires understanding why so many sufferers reject the notion of physical pain resulting from emotional pain. Healing is a choice, like happiness. If you want to see deeper and heal, start absorbing more information on TMS: Tension Myoneural Syndrome, aka, The Mindbody Syndrome.

If a sufferer wants to defend his or her pain, then he or she will find a way to criticize the TMS message. I'll read the misunderstandings after this book is published. The road to hell is indeed paved with the best of intentions. Some will say, "Save your money, there's nothing new here, it's all unproven!" But those same naysayers then need to visit "The TMS Healing Wall of Victory" playlist on YouTube and witness those who have healed from crippling pain, and many other serious health problems with this knowledge. *The proof is in the pudding.*

Finally, for anyone who desires to end their suffering, this information will change your life for the better, forever. You've found your answer. Don't let those who can't understand confuse you and stop you from healing. I KNOW you can heal, and I want to hear your story when you do! I look forward to that day when you have joined the ranks of so many others who have benefited from this great Truth. Thank you John Sarno, doctor.

**Happiness first, and good health will certainly follow ...**

# About The Author

Steve Ozanich, a mindbody health consultant, life-coach and author, penned *The Great Pain Deception* and *Dr. John Sarno's Top 10 Healing Discoveries*, based on his own experience, the work of John Sarno, MD, and ten years of intensive research. Over the past 16 years, Ozanich has helped to teach thousands of people how to heal themselves through his lectures, books, articles, and interviews. Steve is also the author of two children's books. He currently has a restraining order against the emperor.

He earned three degrees from Youngstown State University, AAS, BSAS, and MBA, with four consecutive Distinguished Student Awards from the Williamson School.

In addition to being a mindbody health consultant and life coach, the Ohio-based Ozanich is a health blogger with JenningsWire, a health lecturer, certified personal fitness trainer, acoustic guitar player, and golf swing coach.

# Appendix A

# What can I expect when I see a TMS doctor?

I have often been asked by my readers, "What can I expect when I see a TMS doctor?" So I asked one. The following is the response that I received from Paul Gwozdz, MD, who sees TMS patients in NJ. [Reprinted with permission]

Steve, I have been seeing TMS patients now for close to 16 years and have been pretty much following the same protocol for these patients over that time. It is the protocol that I learned from Dr. Sarno when I trained under him as a doctor in 2001.

During the initial TMS visit I really have two primary goals. One is to reassure myself that the patient does in fact have TMS and secondly to piece together the patient's history so that I can better understand all of the causes of the patient's TMS. While doing so I often times have to determine what the patient's initial TMS presenting symptom was and not just what the current TMS symptom is. The reason is that I want and need to determine all the underlying causes of the TMS. For instance, if the patient's back pain started about the time that their spouse announced that they were leaving the marriage, that gives me a clue as to the underlying cause of their TMS; but if I track their TMS symptoms back to when they were four and they were having a lot of abdominal pain that was causing them to miss school, then I may be able to determine an even more important cause of their TMS. I have found that I can be most effective if I spend 90 minutes in the initial encounter with each patient, so that is what I schedule when the patient calls and requests a TMS appointment.

My belief is that TMS is actually a diagnosis of exclusion. I cannot just look at a patient and examine the patient to determine that they have TMS. I need to hear the history and also prefer to have the reassurance that they have pursued their symptoms with other physical doctors and therefore we have excluded any serious problems such as malignancy. Of course, this is not to say that I will trust the diagnosis provided by the other doctors as the cause of the patient's pain but instead I will interpret the other doctor's diagnosis as Dr. Sarno taught me. Once I have reassured myself that the patient has had a thorough workup, and that they do not have any serious underlying problems, then I am able to provide the assurance that the patient needs in order to be cured of their TMS.

This is important because lack of confidence by the TMS doctor would cause a lack of confidence in the TMS patient, and therefore likely end in a poor result. I always try very hard to be sure in my own mind that the patient does in fact have TMS and I find that spending the extended period of time with the patient usually yields a much better result.

During the initial visit I start out by listening to the patient's history of their physical ailments and trying to understand what was going on in their life when they developed their symptoms. Then I explore their past medical history, past surgical history, family history, childhood history, and explore their relationships with spouse, family, and friends, and then I try to develop a timeline in my own mind linking their stressors to the development of their symptoms in order to determine all the root causes of the TMS symptoms. A standard medical physical exam is completed while concentrating on some of the tender points that tend to be associated with TMS patients, just as Dr. Sarno always did. Although the physical exam is important, your readers should understand that it really is the thorough psychosocial and medical history that is critical to the diagnosis of the TMS patient.

As I said, I feel more confident diagnosing a patient with TMS if they have had thorough medical workups by other specialists such as neurologists or orthopedic surgeons. This allows me to be sure that I am not missing a medical/physical cause of their pain. An MRI or CT of the affected area is also required before I see the patient in order to be sure that I am not missing anything else.

After the patient has completed the 90-minute initial exam with me and I have determined that they have TMS, I invite them back for my two to three-hour lecture. The lecture is also an important part of the treatment of the patient. I model my lecture very much after the lecture that Dr. Sarno did except that I have added some additional information, particularly regarding the symptom imperative and all the different symptoms that TMS patients can have. I believe this is very important because I do not want the TMS patient to be relieved of their presenting symptom only to find out that because of the symptom imperative they now have some new symptom and do not realize that it, too, is just TMS.

In the first part of the lecture we talk about all the different symptoms that a TMS patient can have. We then discuss some specifics regarding back pain for those patients with back pain, though many of my TMS patients do not have back pain. We then review the physiology of TMS. This is important because the TMS patient needs to understand how it is that the emotional brain can actually cause their symptom. Up until this point the patient most likely was led to believe that their abnormality found on an x-ray or MRI was the cause of their symptom; not that their emotional mind was creating the symptom as a distraction to keep them from thinking about the things they don't want to think about. Understanding the physiology can help the patient to convince themselves that emotional issues can cause physical pain.

In part two of the lecture, we discuss the emotional mind. We discuss three primary areas of our emotions that lead to TMS: difficulties in our childhood, our personality traits, and current-day stressors. We then are ready to launch into an approach to cure ourselves of TMS. It is my belief that there are many different approaches that can be useful for curing TMS. A number of TMS authors have put out very good books suggesting a number of different approaches. I believe that each of these approaches can work very well for select patients. Not every approach will work for every patient. I teach an approach that I used for myself and I've used for my patients over the years and that is just simply creating the list of sources of your TMS and then talking to your brain throughout the day reminding yourself that it is not physical causes that are the cause of your TMS, but rather, the causes are the items on your list. The patient is then given a four-page homework assignment modeled after the one that Dr. Sarno used and the patient is sent home for one month to do their homework and eliminate all of their TMS symptoms. At the end of the month the patient is asked to come back to the office in order to review their progress and if the patient has not been successful, to determine why not. I do find it very important to do the monthly follow up as it often times results in an unsuccessful patient becoming successful. I help the patient to tweak what they are saying to their brains and how they are saying it. We compare the list that the patient developed as part of the homework with the list that I developed as part of the initial visit, to be sure that all the sources of TMS are covered.

If the patient is not cured after two or three months then the patient will be referred to one of the several TMS psychotherapists that I work with.

I should also mention here that in the lecture I frequently encourage patients to raise their questions and challenges. I want all the patients to completely understand what I'm talking about and not leave my office with any unresolved questions or concerns that might lead to them not being cured. If I don't know the answer, I will admit to that fact; but in most cases I can eliminate their concern, which should help to result in a more rapid cure. Patients are not required to speak; this is not a group therapy session but does occasionally change into one.

Some patients can cure themselves by reading, while others need the additional help of a TMS doctor to provide the confidence that their pain is TMS. I know that in 1987, I needed Dr. Sarno's reassurance when I was an engineering manager, not a doctor; now I am in a position to be able to provide that same care. I always credit Dr. Sarno for giving me back my life and wish to share the knowledge that we are healthy human beings who do not need to be in pain.

Dr. Gwozdz' website: www.gwozdzmd.com

# Appendix B

# Some Dr. Sarno Success Stories

Dr. Sarno retired from medicine in April of 2012 after a 50-year career that was injected with bewildering controversy, but with a much greater dose of hope. He planted a legacy that will certainly grow forever as long as the light continues to shine on it. The good doctor helped so many people heal that many are now established in careers that center around his work. One example is the Peer Review Network TMSWiki.org that was born both out of the desire to help TMS sufferers using Dr. Sarno's work, and as a means to thank him for all that he contributed to humanity's health. Other examples are the Pain Psychology Center led by Executive Director Alan Gordon, LCSW, in California, and SIRPA, created by pain-specialist Georgie Oldfield, MCSP, in the United Kingdom.

Anyone can visit TMSWiki.org for free, as well as the Facebook page, "A Page Honoring John E. Sarno, MD" to both seek help and to read the thank you notes that steadily come in from around the world. The TMSWiki may first appear daunting but it's fairly user-friendly. I chose a few Dr. Sarno "back pain" thank you notes from the "Thank You, Dr. Sarno" page in order to provide a few more examples of how magnificently the TMS process works (reprinted with permission, photos removed for privacy consideration).

The anecdotal stories are the most important proof that Dr. Sarno is correct, and that he has been all along. I've added them to the Appendices to help people see the effects of his work. I do not know, nor have I ever met any of these former sufferers. But I understand exactly how they feel ....

### JH's Thank You

Dear Dr. Sarno:

In 2000, my back had deteriorated to the point where walking over ten steps was practically impossible. I spent considerable time and money engaged with the "cures" of the day: yoga, chiropractors, acupuncture, rolfing, prolotherapy, etc. Nothing helped. I therefore underwent surgery to correct the diagnosed problem of spinal stenosis. My surgery was deemed a success; within six months I was ambulatory again. It felt good. My instructions were clear: no heavy lifting, bend a certain way, don't put too much pressure on your back, etc.

About one and a half years later, I started to experience my initial symptoms all over again. The "pins and needles" feeling in my legs returned, accompanied by pain and numbness. I could feel that within a month's time, I'd be back walking like Groucho Marx. I felt hopeless, depressed and desperate. I got lucky: someone casually mentioned your name and to check out your books. In the Amazon reviews, I encountered a positive reviewer whose diagnosis was the same as mine. I ditched all of my advisors (you gotta call this new chiropractor, he's amazing!) and committed myself to your concepts, memorizing them and carrying them around with me. I stopped all attempts at having someone else "fix" me. That was one of the more difficult things that I have ever done.

Approximately three months later, my back pain had ceased. It took about another year or two to conquer the fear of lifting things, but I did it. I've had a few TMS equivalents along the way, but thinking psychologically has given me a new lease on life. I'm profoundly grateful for all of your insights and research. Your work continues to have a large influence on my life—thank you for truly opening my eyes!

Sincerely,

JH

## KO's Thank You

I was living in NYC, working in film production, and running 15–20 miles a week. Magazine articles warned about running on pavement and advised making sure there was enough support in running shoes. I never had a hint of a problem until one day on a particularly stressful shoot I was impatiently hauling an ice chest from one part of the set to the other, and it happened. I pulled a muscle in my back. The next morning I felt an electric-like jolt when I leaned over the sink to brush my teeth, followed by an incredibly painful muscle spasm that dropped me to my knees. When I could move again I called a friend who recommended a physical therapist. She listened to my story and told me I had probably herniated a disc and that the "electric" feeling was caused by the disc impinging on my sciatic nerve. I could picture it. My back kept spasming. I took muscle relaxers that made my tongue thick and uncooperative. The sciatica hurt, and I took pain pills that would have knocked out a horse. I slept on a mat on our hard wood floor. Nothing worked. Over the next few months the sciatica crept down my leg and finally reached all the way into my heel which became tingly and numb.

As it went from bad to worse, I went to chiropractors. I got Rolfed(TM). I got acupuncture. I got acupuncture with pulses of electricity running through it. I went to back specialists recommended by heads of athletic departments. I was X-rayed, CAT

Scanned, and MRI'd. I learned I have scoliosis, extensive arthritic degeneration of my bottom five vertebrae, and several more slightly herniated discs that would surely cripple me if nothing was done. In any event, I was advised never to run again. The pain had become so bad, I couldn't walk more than three or four feet without tearing up. I couldn't sit upright, so I worked lying on my back. I slept with my right knee propped on hard pillows. A very expensive specialist with a posh office overlooking Columbus Circle told me I might never walk again if I didn't have surgery immediately.

A producer I met gave me a copy of Dr. Sarno's book "Mind Over Back Pain." I was insulted. I didn't accept the idea that this kind of pain was in my head. I had cat scans, MRIs, and an x-ray that showed the horrific problems in my spine. If I touched the place where the herniated disc was impinging on the nerve, the pain was so intense it made me nauseous. But I was terrified of back surgery going wrong. I wanted to run again. So I read the book. Cover to cover. It was encouraging. It made sense. I hoped it was true, but I wasn't sure. I mentioned Dr. Sarno to the last back doctor I will ever see. He hadn't read the book, but he'd heard of Dr. Sarno, and he scoffed at the mind-body connection in a smug way that I found offensive. So I called Dr. Sarno's office to make an appointment to see the man himself. I was told he didn't take many patients, and that the waiting list was months long. I begged. I pleaded. I somehow convinced his secretary to put me on the phone with him.

Dr. Sarno: "This is John Sarno."

Me: "Dr. Sarno, thank you for taking my call. I read your book and I think I'm a Sarno patient, but I need to see you to be sure."

Dr. Sarno: "You should read the book again instead."

Me: "You don't understand, I've ... (and here I listed what I'd been through) ... and I just need to be sure there's really nothing wrong with my back."

Dr. Sarno: "There's nothing wrong with your back."

Me: "I just need to see you in person."

Dr. Sarno: "I'm not charismatic. I'm not going to 'heal' you."

Me: "Please, if you could just see me so I can be sure."

Dr. Sarno: "Young lady, it's very expensive. And I don't take insurance."

Me (sensing he was going to give in): "That's fine!"

Dr. Sarno: (audible sigh) "Okay. I'll put you back on with my secretary."

She had a cancellation for the next day. My husband carried me through the halls of NYU hospital to Dr. Sarno's small waiting room where I lay on the floor. When he called my name, I raised myself with my hands underneath me, crawled into his office front-wise, and lowered myself gingerly onto the floor next to the chair that was there. He peered over the desk at me. A small man with salt and pepper hair and black glasses, he gestured impatiently at the chair, "Aren't you going to sit?"

"I can't," I said and my tears started to roll.

"So you read my book?" he asked.

"Yes, twice," I said.

"I have a new one coming out. I advise writing down everything that's upsetting you. What do you do for a living?"

"I work in film production."

He groaned. "You don't know how many of you people I get in here." I could see he was taking notes.

I had brought my scans in big envelopes. I asked him if he wanted to see them. He said no. I asked, "How do you KNOW there's nothing wrong with my back?"

He waved his hand dismissively at the envelopes I offered, "You wouldn't have been able to crawl in here like a crab if there was anything wrong with your back."

I said, "But there's a place there that hurts so much when I touch it, it makes me want to vomit."

He lowered his glasses and looked over the desk at me, "Don't touch it."

I thought about that for a second. "Don't you even want to examine me?"

"Okay." He seemed resigned. He stood up and opened a door behind him that connected to a small examining room. As I scooted on hands and feet toward the room, I told him my leg was numb along the back and down to the heel. Once I had made my way up onto the table, he did a needle test on the back of my leg and confirmed, "You're right. It's numb."

"Doesn't that mean anything?"

"No." He repeated some of the facts about TMS and how the symptoms develop that I recalled from his book. He told me he'd written a new book incorporating what he'd learned since he'd written the first one. I started to believe him.

I made myself stand up and walk out. The whole thing had taken 15 minutes.

In the waiting room I leaned on my amazed husband. It was painful. But I was standing, and walking.

"By the way," Dr. Sarno said from his office door, "don't sleep with a pillow under your knee anymore." I hadn't mentioned the pillows.

The pain and numbness took several months to go completely away, but my recovery started that day. There was nothing wrong with my back. Patients of Dr. Sarno were encouraged to attend a class he taught about the mind-body connection and how we needed to reinforce the association between chronic pain and life stresses. I took the class.

I saw a therapist, briefly. I filled notebook after notebook with lists of things that were making me angry, scaring me, and upsetting me. I listed the same things over and over again. I was never going to be able to change most of them, but acknowledging them, driving the association between the things on the list and the pain into my subconscious finally ended my ordeal.

I still get what I call "Sarno Things." It's my personality. At stressful times I've had mock arthritis, mock bursitis, mock "runner's knee," mock TMJ, mock carpal tunnel, mock plantar faciitis. As soon as I realize what is happening, I stop and make myself list everything that's bothering me. If I'm running, I ignore the pain and make the lists in my head. And every time the pain goes away like a headache fades when you take ibuprofen.

I know I will never have chronic pain again. I don't pay money to masseuses or chiropractors. I don't worry about running on cement, or the shape of my running shoes. I run 20 to 30 miles a week. My life is my own, thanks to you, Dr. John Sarno. For as long as I live I will be grateful to you.

I hope you enjoy your retirement.

All the very best,

K.O.

## Michele's Thank You

Dear Dr. Sarno,

Thank you does not even come close to acknowledging how much I appreciate all you have done for me. For 15 years, I lived with ever more frequent back spasms and the fear of never knowing when they would happen again. My life was so compromised that I missed out on many opportunities with my family and career. You gave me back the joy of living in six weeks by just reading a book (*Healing Back Pain*). Before that, I believed that I was doomed to a life of pain because of my so-called structural defects. It was miraculous. I have since returned to school, got my master's degree in counseling and presently work as a mindbody TMS therapist.

I am so in awe of your perseverance and bravery in believing TMS to be a mindbody condition. It had to be so difficult to be treated as an outcast in your own profession and still stay true to your beliefs.

I wish you all the best in your retirement.

With deepest gratitude,

Michele

## J.N.'s Thank You

Dr. Sarno, your books have saved me time and time again for the last 12 years. Back in 2000, I was suffering from multiple food sensitivities, multiple chemical sensitivity, and unidentified pelvic pain. I'd tried everything, and had had to quit my job due to a coworker's aftershave and find another place to work. Then, I started getting low back pain, and found your book "Healing Back Pain." It intrigued me, and I bought "The MindBody Prescription." I read the book cover to cover, over and over again. My back pain disappeared within two months. It dawned on me that my pelvic pain was TMS, and that disappeared soon thereafter. It was harder for me to accept that my food and chemical sensitivities were TMS, but they also disappeared.

Over the years, I have repeatedly adopted manifestations of TMS, and time and time again, I have reread your book and have eliminated the symptoms of the great majority of them (and reduced a few others, so far). I'm deeply grateful to you and your work, Dr. Sarno. Thank you from the bottom of my heart for all you've done. Please enjoy your retirement and know how many hearts and lives you've touched. Much much love!!!!

-J. N.

## Hasanna's Thank You

Dear Dr. Sarno,

I'm so happy to have this opportunity to say thank you. Your wonderful work has changed my life personally and professionally. Twelve years ago, I had already had two (unnecessary!) shoulder surgeries and I was starting to have severe hip pain when I discovered your book *Healing Back Pain.* Within a month the hip pain, as well as chronic back and neck pain, were gone. And as a TMS psychotherapist, I've been able to help so many other people get their lives back, too. Thank you for persevering for so long in the face of so much resistance!

Hasanna

## Allan's Thank You

I am now 82. At 70 years of age I became progressively worse in terms of back pain. It was diagnosed as spinal stenosis. I lost most of my strength in both legs which was diagnosed as being caused by motor nerve impingement from the spinal stenosis. I walked with a cane and then only for a few feet at a time before the pain became too intense. I was anticipating that I might spend the rest of my life in a wheel chair. My son sent me Dr. Sarno's book which I devoured. I read it over and over. This was the summer of 2000. The pain left. My strength returned. The pain never came back.

I sent a letter of appreciation to Dr. Sarno. I have his reply of October 19, 2000 framed on my wall.

Allan

## Ben's Thank You

Dear Dr. Sarno,

Reading your books felt like awaking from a very bad dream. Thanks to you, I am not having nightmares anymore. You did not only help me with my pain, but you also greatly improved my terrible MS relapses. You have also shown me, how to see my true self and how to change myself into a better person, a loving husband and a future father.

You dedicated your life to helping people, with the majority of your colleagues not believing in you. The sacrifices you made for helping and curing us will be remembered.

The picture was taken before I got TMS. Thanks to you, I can go back now and take pictures like that again.

Thank you Benjamin

## Panda's Thank You

Dear Dr. Sarno,

I wanted to write and say thank you for totally transforming my life with your work on TMS. Before I knew about TMS I spent 10 years in severe and debilitating back pain and couldn't walk more than about 100 yards without being in agony.

After reading *Healing Back Pain* I finally had hope and within six months I was walking more and more without pain. This is a recent photo of me and my family at the ice rink. I have learned to figure skate and am doing jumps and spins, I still can't believe I can do so much these days; I am so grateful to you for giving me my life back. I can never thank you enough,

Panda

## Colleen's Thank You

Dear Dr. Sarno,

Your contribution to the betterment of my life began well over a decade ago. I was a young woman who had suffered from lower back pain since my teenage years. I went to many doctors and chiropractors hoping for a solution and was told over and over again that I should focus on strengthening my abs. I would just shake my head in bewilderment because none of those doctors had ever asked me what I did for a living ... at that time I was an aerobics instructor and personal fitness trainer! There was NOTHING weak about my abs! So I just knew that medical science did not have the answer to my problem.

When my trusted family physician suggested that the next step was spinal surgery, my intuition kicked in high gear and I knew in my gut that the answer was out there somewhere, and it wasn't surgery.

Someone had mentioned your book, *The Mind Body Prescription* to me years ago. I read it, and found myself in those pages. It was easy for me because I have every personality trait associated with TMS. There was no doubt in my mind that this was my problem.

I was pain-free after that for quite a while, but I didn't have the often spoken about "book cure." My pain does come back in different places now from time to time, but it serves as my reminder to slow down, to not take life so seriously, to put into practice better forms of self-care. I have a new and completely different relationship to pain now.

I went back to school, received my Master's Degree in Psychology, and now help others who suffer from TMS in my private practice.

Through me you continue to heal those that suffer from chronic pain. Thank you for your courage and dedication to bringing your paradigm-shifting views to the world. You are a maverick and an inspiration to us all.

With Gratitude,
Colleen, MFT

## Mark's Thank You

Dear Dr. Sarno,

I am so glad to have this opportunity to thank you, because it is something I have been meaning to do for twenty years! My back pain started at age 32, and I had episodes of severe pain and back spasms that left me flat on my back in bed or on the floor for three days at a time. I remember crawling to the bathroom because I couldn't bear the indignity of using a bedpan. That's how bad it was. I pretty much gave up my active lifestyle of running and playing basketball. My sister also suffered from back pain, probably worse than mine. Fortunately for her (and for me) as a last resort before surgery she went to see you, and reported her success to me. She then sent me a Xerox copy of your book, and within days I was on my way to a complete "cure." So many of my severe symptoms were directly addressed in your book. My first episode was triggered by a sneeze while I was bent over and putting on a sock. I remember many times looking in the mirror and gasping at how crooked I looked. I am now 58 and have been pain-free and active for over 20 years! It has truly been wonderful. All because of you.

At times I have felt a little guilty because I had been helped so dramatically by someone (you) and I hadn't even bought your book! I have since purchased multiple copies of several of your books mainly to lend to friends who are suffering from back pain. I have tried to share my success with others with mixed results. It is very frustrating to see people suffering and going to chiropractors and acupuncturists and surgeons and drug dispensers while somehow being unwilling to accept the simple solution.

But for me, it has been one of the best things that has happened in my life and has really allowed me to enjoy my life to the fullest.

Thank you!

Best regards,

Mark

## K's Thank You

Dear Dr. Sarno,

Words could never, ever express how grateful I am to have found you. I think my body always knew you were right. My awareness just had to catch up.

I had back pain for 25+ years. I was told my pain was from scoliosis and myofascial pain syndrome. I tried to find relief through Tylenol, chiropractors, physical therapy, and lifting light weights at the gym. Coinciding with my back pain for all those years was TMJ and headaches. They pounded and pounded, mostly during a stressful day at work. I did more PT, used a TENS unit, moist heat, tried acupuncture, and lifted weights more. Even if the pain subsided for a very brief time, it always came back.

Then, somehow, I found *Healing Back Pain*. It sounded just like me, I couldn't believe it. Then I read *The Mindbody Prescription* and I related to that one even more. I made an appointment to see you; I knew I had TMS, but I had to hear it from you.

Thank you for changing my life. It is no longer ruled by pain every day. I have no limitations and that is incredibly liberating. I admire you for telling it like it is and for staying true to your convictions.

I will never forget you. I hope you have a long and happy retirement. I will miss you.

With gratitude forever,

K

## Michael's Thank You

Dear Dr. Sarno,

As a second year medical student, I began to experience back pain for the first time in my life. I serendipitously came across your work and it changed my life forever. You taught me the greatest lesson I ever learned in medicine: to cure disease, you must treat the cause. Symptomatic treatment is poor medicine. You also introduced me to the powerful and fascinating realm of psychosomatic medicine, which is the missing dimension in so many of the diagnoses we as physicians encounter today.

I could never thank you enough for what you have given me. You are my mentor and hero in medicine and anything I ever achieve professionally will be because of you. You dedicated your career to patient care, which speaks volumes to the type of person that you are. You have healed tens of thousands of patients in your office and millions more through your books. You knew you were right, but decided that it was more important to spend your time curing people than proving all the nonbelievers wrong through research that would never satisfy or change them anyway. You put your patients before your ego and kudos to you for doing that.

Thanks for inviting me to one of your patient panel sessions a few years ago. It was a dream come true to finally see you in person. For the record, I have never had any back pain since reading your books. That isn't to say that new TMS equivalents don't pop up from time to time, but they too are easily squashed once I put my mind to it. You have armed me with powerful tools to live a healthier and happier life and to empower patients, friends, and family to do the same.

The story has only begun. There is now an army of young physicians and researchers who are intent on preserving your legacy and continuing your work for decades to come. I am certain that when all is said and done and we look back on the history of psychosomatic medicine that your name will be right next to those of Freud, Breuer, Alexander, and others who have left a lasting impression on this field.

I wish you the happiest and healthiest of retirements. You have certainly earned it.

Thank you, Dr. Sarno!

Michael

## Laura's Thank You

Dear Dr. Sarno,

You certainly changed my life for the better in so many ways!

I was 33 years old and the mother of two daughters, ages 15 months and 6 months of age, when "out of the blue," I began to suffer excruciating lower back pain/sciatica– worse pain than the two natural childbirths I had recently experienced.

I found your book "Mind Over Back Pain" and immediately booked an appointment with you at NYU's Rusk Institute.

Within a month my back pain was gone.

Over the years I've had other TMS symptoms – shoulder/neck pain, and foot pain, for example, and sometimes it took me a while to realize that this new pain was just another manifestation of my old syndrome.

I think of any new pain symptom as my personal canary in the coal mine– alerting me that I am getting too close to the edge of my emotional comfort zone.

Your work not only gave me a life free of chronic pain and possible addiction to pain medications, but it also opened my mind to many other facets of mind/body medicine and emotional wellness.

I have traveled the world and enjoyed an active life all because of you– here is a photo of my husband Russ and me at the Great Wall of China in 2011!

I am eternally grateful! You are an amazing human being.

Thank you!

Laura

## Dustin's Thank You

Dear Dr. Sarno,

In my late teens I began a 10-year journey of one physical ailment after another and it continued until I studied your work. It started with knee pain, mild carpel tunnel syndrome, then lower back pain, severe allergies, asthma, pancreatitis and finished off with severe ulcerative colitis, all with no known cause and most with no known cure other than surgery for a couple of them. I tried cortisone shots in my knee, braces and therapy for my knee and wrist, inhalers and nasal spray for allergies and asthma, stretches and chiropractors for my back, a wheelbarrow of pills, juicing, fasting, and diet changes for colitis. I even had a visit at one of the top four hospitals in the United States in search of help for pancreatitis and colitis only to come home with no answers. I was at a loss. In my mind, being in my mid-20s, I should have been at the peak of health.

As a long time listener of Howard Stern, I heard him mention you several times over the years but always about back pain. I dismissed it because I only had a brief encounter with it but one day he went a little deeper and touched on the mindbody connection. It triggered something and I bought all of your books. I'm now almost 31, take no medication and I'm in the best health of my life. My breathing tests since studying your work have been "perfect" the pulmonologist says and he has taken me off all inhalers. The allergies remain but have been reduced by 90 percent.

During the time period I was studying your work I had an accident and suffered a Type 4 AC shoulder separation. After I healed up through physical therapy and was feeling great, I put your theory of pain returning to the site of an old injury to the test. I randomly started feeling a severe pain in my shoulder as if someone was trying to drive a nail into it, it did not follow suit to what I had been doing physically and I "talked myself out of it." The pain tried a couple more times to come back, I immediately shut it down and it hasn't returned. I can't thank you enough and as everyone else says, I am forever in debt to you, Dr. Sarno.

THANK YOU!!

Dustin

The thank yous to Dr. Sarno go on and on. Even today, retired and in his 90s he continues to receive a tremendous amount of email thank yous. And yet, many say that what he discovered can't be done ....

The PPD/TMS Peer Network (PTPN) is a 501(c)(3) nonprofit organization founded in 2009. We seek to relieve suffering from Tension Myositis Syndrome (TMS) by raising awareness, providing information based on scientific evidence, facilitating expression of a wide variety of perspectives, and giving individual support to people with TMS. Like many others, we suffered from terrible pain and other symptoms for many years before learning about this approach. All the members of our organization suffered from TMS at some point in their lives, and the majority of these members consider themselves to have recovered from chronic pain and now experience little to no pain. Source: TMSWiki.org

# Appendix C

# 5 Regrets of Dying People

**Listed are the five most common regrets of people on their death bed, as compiled by former hospice worker Bronnie Ware[82]. They are very similar to the sentiments I have witnessed from those folks who experience back pain.**
**Note #1, #3 and #5.**

1. I wish I'd had the courage to live a life true to myself, not the life others expected of me.

2. I wish I hadn't worked so hard.

3. I wish I'd had the courage to express my feelings.

4. I wish I had stayed in touch with my friends.

5. I wish I had let myself be happier.

# Appendix D

# Faulty Pain Diagnoses

Some of the more common and ludicrous professional diagnoses which were later proven to be TMS are listed below.

- You have an unstable spine.
- You have low back pain because your spine is similar in shape to a chimpanzee's.
- You need to sit a certain way.
- You have bone on bone.
- Your mattress is too soft.
- You pinched a nerve.
- Your ligaments are too tight.
- You have piriformis syndrome.
- You have one leg that is longer than the other.
- Your knee and shoulder need to be scoped out.
- You have fibromyalgia "disease."
- Your discs, stenosis, arthritis, and crooked spine are causing your pain.
- You slipped a spinal disc.
- Your eyes are too narrow.
- Your bladder is too small.
- Your leg is longer than the other as a result of uneven hips (pelvic obliquity).
- Your spine is weak.
- You have to lose weight to heal.
- You need a knee replacement.
- Your tendon is too short.
- Your rotator cuff needs surgery—or you will lose the use of your arm.
- Your cervical vertebrae are straight instead of being "curly."
- Your iPod is causing you pain (bad iPosture).
- You have bad Achilles' heel tendons and will need to walk only on level surfaces, the rest of your life.
- You sneezed and herniated five discs.

- You have text-neck.

- You have Dormant Butt Syndrome (weak glutes)

- You wear the wrong type of jeans *(comment made by a chief spine surgeon in New York).*

- Your back hurts because you have ghetto-booty *(yes, this is a real diagnosis made by a Tennessee physician for back pain).*

**Insanity repeating itself everyday ... this list will certainly grow as the search for the "cure" needlessly continues.**

# Appendix E

# Brinjikji et al. Meta-Analysis of Spine Imaging Studies

Systematic Literature Review of Imaging Features of Spinal Degeneration in Asymptomatic Populations. 814 Brinjikji Apr 2015 www.ajnr.org
Source: SPINE, http://dx.doi.org/10.3174/ajnr.A4173
W. Brinjikji, P.H. Luetmer, B. Comstock, B.W. Bresnahan, L.E. Chen, R.A. Deyo, S. Halabi, J.A. Turner, A.L. Avins, K. James, J.T. Wald, D.F. Kallmes, and J.G. Jarvik.

Jarvik JG, Deyo RA. Diagnostic evaluation of low back pain with emphasis on imaging. Ann Intern Med 2002; 137:586–97.

Deyo RA, Cherkin D, Conrad D, et al. Cost, controversy, crisis: low back pain and the health of the public. Annu Rev Public Health 1991; 12:141–56.

Li AL, Yen D. Effect of increased MRI and CT scan utilization on clinical decision-making in patients referred to a surgical clinic for back pain. Can J Surg 2011; 54:128–32.

Carragee E, Alamin T, Cheng I, et al. Are first-time episodes of serious LBP associated with new MRI findings? Spine J 2006; 6: 624–35.

Boden SD, Davis DO, Dina TS, et al. Abnormal magnetic-resonance scans of the lumbar spine in asymptomatic subjects: a prospective investigation. J Bone Joint Surg Am 1990; 72:403–08.

Kalichman L, Kim DH, Li L, et al. Computed tomography-evaluated features of spinal degeneration: prevalence, intercorrelation, and association with self-reported low back pain. Spine J 2010; 10:200–08.

Wiesel SW, Tsourmas N, Feffer HL, et al. A study of computer-assisted tomography. I. The incidence of positive CAT scans in an asymptomatic group of patients. Spine[3](Phila Pa 1976) 1984; 9: 549–51.

Fardon DF, Milette PC. Nomenclature and classification of lumbar disc pathology: recommendations of the combined task forces of the North American Spine Society, American Society of Spine Radiology, and American Society of Neuroradiology. Spine (Phila Pa 1976) 2001; 26:E93–E113.

Sasiadek MJ, Bladowska J. Imaging of degenerative spine disease– the state of the art. Adv Clin Exp Med 2012; 21:133–42.

Berg L, Hellum C, Gjertsen O, et al. Do more MRI findings imply worse disability or more intense low back pain? A cross-sectional study of candidates for lumbar disc prosthesis. Skeletal Radiol 2013; 42:1593–602.

Takatalo J, Karppinen J, Niinima¨ki J, et al. Association of Modic
    changes, Schmorl's nodes, spondylolytic defects, high-intensity
    zone lesions, disc herniations, and radial tears with low back
    symptom severity among young Finnish adults. Spine (Phila Pa
    1976) 2012; 37:1231–39.

Steffens D, Hancock MJ, Maher CG, et al. Does magnetic resonance
    imaging predict future low back pain? A systematic review. Eur J
    Pain 2014;18: 755–65.

Kovacs FM, Arana E, Royuela A, et al. Vertebral endplate changes are
    not associated with chronic low back pain among Southern
    European subjects: a case control study. AJNR Am J Neuroradiol
    2012;33: 1519–24.

Kaneoka K, Shimizu K, Hangai M, et al. Lumbar intervertebral disk
    degeneration in elite competitive swimmers: a case control study.
    Am J Sports Med 2007; 35:1341–45.

Kraft CN, Pennekamp PH, Becker U, et al. Magnetic resonance imaging
    findings of the lumbar spine in elite horseback riders: correlations
    with back pain, body mass index, trunk/leg-length coefficient, and
    riding discipline. Am J Sports Med 2009; 37:2205–13.

Modic MT, Obuchowski NA, Ross JS, et al. Acute low back pain and
    radiculopathy: MR imaging findings and their prognostic role and
    effect on outcome. Radiology 2005; 237:597–604.

Chou R, Fu R, Carrino JA, et al. Imaging strategies for low-back pain:
    systematic review and meta-analysis. Lancet 2009; 373: 463–72.

Carlisle E, Luna M, Tsou PM, et al. Percent spinal canal compromise on
    MRI utilized for predicting the need for surgical treatment in single-
    level lumbar intervertebral disc herniation. Spine J 2005; 5:608–14.

Lurie JD, Moses RA, Tosteson AN, et al. Magnetic resonance imaging
    predictors of surgical outcome in patients with lumbar
    intervertebral disc herniation. Spine (Phila Pa 1976) 2013; 38:1216–
    25.

Greenberg JO, Schnell RG. Magnetic resonance imaging of the lumbar
    spine in asymptomatic adults: cooperative study—American Society
    of Neuroimaging. J Neuroimaging 1991; 1:2–7.

Teraguchi M, Yoshimura N, Hashizume H, et al. Prevalence and
    distribution of intervertebral disc degeneration over the entire spine
    in a population-based cohort: the Wakayama Spine Study.
    Osteoarthritis Cartilage 2014; 22:104–10.

Jarvik JJ, Hollingworth W, Heagerty P, et al. The Longitudinal
    Assessment of Imaging and Disability of the Back (LAIDBack) study:
    baseline data. Spine (Phila Pa 1976) 2001; 26:1158–66.

Jarvik JG, Hollingworth W, Heagerty PJ, et al. Three-year incidence of
    low back pain in an initially asymptomatic cohort: clinical and
    imaging risk factors. Spine (Phila Pa 1976) 2005; 30:1541–48;
    discussion 1549.

Arana E, Kovacs FM, Royuela A, et al. Influence of nomenclature in the interpretation of lumbar disk contour on MR imaging: a comparison of the agreement using the combined task force and the Nordic nomenclatures. AJNR Am J Neuroradiol 2011; 32:1143–48.

Arana E, Royuela A, Kovacs FM, et al. Lumbar spine: agreement in the interpretation of 1.5-TMRimages by using the Nordic Modic Consensus Group classification form. Radiology 2010; 254:809–17.

Thornton A, Lee P. Publication bias in meta-analysis: its causes and consequences. J Clin Epidemiol 2000; 53:207–16.

Boden SD, Riew KD, Yamaguchi K, et al. Orientation of the lumbar facet joints: association with degenerative disc disease. J Bone Joint Surg Am 1996; 78:403–11.

Boos N, Rieder R, Schade V, et al. 1995 Volvo Award in clinical sciences: the diagnostic accuracy of magnetic resonance imaging, work perception, and psychosocial factors in identifying symptomatic disc herniations. Spine (Phila Pa 1976) 1995; 20: 2613–25.

Capel A, Medina FS, Medina D, et al. Magnetic resonance study of lumbar disks in female dancers. Am J Sports Med 2009; 37:1208–13.

Danielson B, Willen J. Axially loaded magnetic resonance image of the lumbar spine in asymptomatic individuals. Spine (Phila Pa 1976) 2001; 26:2601–06.

Dora C, Walchli B, Elfering A, et al. The significance of spinal canal dimensions in discriminating symptomatic from asymptomatic disc herniations. Eur Spine J 2002; 11:575–81.

Edmondston SJ, Song S, Bricknell RV, et al. MRI evaluation of lumbar spine flexion and extension in asymptomatic individuals. Man Ther 2000; 5:158–64.

Erkintalo MO, Salminen JJ, Alanen AM, et al. Development of degenerative changes in the lumbar intervertebral disk: results of a prospective MR imaging study in adolescents with and without low-back pain. Radiology 1995; 196:529–33.

Feng T, Zhao P, Liang G. Clinical significance on protruded nucleus pulposus: a comparative study of 44 patients with lumbar intervertebral disc protrusion and 73 asymptomatic controls in tridimentional computed tomography [in Chinese]. Zhongguo Zhong Xi Yi Jie He Za Zhi 2000; 20:347–49.

Gibson MJ, Szypryt EP, Buckley JH, et al. Magnetic resonance imaging of adolescent disc herniation. J Bone Joint Surg Br 1987; 69:699–703.

Hamanishi C, Kawabata T, Yosii T, et al. Schmorl's nodes on magnetic resonance imaging. Their incidence and clinical relevance. Spine (Phila Pa 1976) 1994; 19:450–53.

Healy JF, Healy BB, Wong WH, et al. Cervical and lumbar MRI in asymptomatic older male lifelong athletes: frequency of degenerative findings. J Comput Assist Tomogr 1996; 20:107–12.

Jensen MC, Brant-Zawadzki MN, Obuchowski N, et al. Magnetic resonance imaging of the lumbar spine in people without back pain. N Engl J Med 1994; 331:69–73.

Kanayama M, Togawa D, Takahashi C, et al. Cross-sectional magnetic resonance imaging study of lumbar disc degeneration in 200 healthy individuals. J Neurosurg Spine 2009; 11:501–07.

Karakida O, Ueda H, Ueda M, et al. Diurnal T2 value changes in the lumbar intervertebral discs. Clin Radiol 2003; 58:389–92.

Kjaer P, Leboeuf-Yde C, Korsholm L, et al. Magnetic resonance imaging and low back pain in adults: a diagnostic imaging study of 40-year-old men and women. Spine (Phila Pa 1976) 2005; 30:1173–80.

Kovacs FM, Arana E, Royuela A, et al. Disc degeneration and chronic low back pain: an association which becomes nonsignificant when endplate changes and disc contour are taken into account. Neuroradiology 2014; 56:25–33.

Matsumoto M, Okada E, Toyama Y, et al. Tandem age-related lumbar and cervical intervertebral disc changes in asymptomatic subjects. Eur Spine J 2013; 22:708–13.

Paajanen H, Erkintalo M, Parkkola R, et al. Age-dependent correlation of low-back pain and lumbar disc degeneration. Arch Orthop Trauma Surg 1997; 116:106–07.

Paajanen H, Erkintalo M, Kuusela T, et al. Magnetic resonance study of disc degeneration in young low-back pain patients. Spine 1989; 14:982–85.

Ranson CA, Kerslake RW, Burnett AF, et al. Magnetic resonance imaging of the lumbar spine in asymptomatic professional fast bowlers in cricket. J Bone Joint Surg Br 2005; 87:1111–16.

Savage RA, Whitehouse GH, Roberts N. The relationship between the magnetic resonance imaging appearance of the lumbar spine and low back pain, age and occupation in males. Eur Spine J 1997; 6:106–14.

AJNR Am J Neuroradiol 36:811–16 Apr 2015 www.ajnr.org 815.

Silcox DH 3rd, Horton WC, Silverstein AM. MRI of lumbar intervertebral discs: diurnal variations in signal intensities. Spine (Phila Pa 1976) 1995; 20:807–11; discussion 811–12.

Stadnik TW, Lee RR, Coen HL, et al. Annular tears and disk herniation: prevalence and contrast enhancement onMRimages in the absence of low back pain or sciatica. Radiology 1998; 206:49–55.

Szypryt EP, Twining P, Mulholland RC, et al. The prevalence of disc degeneration associated with neural arch defects of the lumbar spine assessed by magnetic resonance imaging. Spine (Phila Pa 1976) 1989; 14:977–81.

Weinreb JC, Wolbarsht LB, Cohen JM, et al. Prevalence of lumbosacral intervertebral disk abnormalities on MR images in pregnant and asymptomatic nonpregnant women. Radiology 1989; 170: 125–28.

Weishaupt D, Zanetti M, Hodler J, et al. MR imaging of the lumbar spine: prevalence of intervertebral disk extrusion and sequestration, nerve root compression, end plate abnormalities, and osteoarthritis of the facet joints in asymptomatic volunteers. Radiology 1998; 209:661–66.

Zobel BB, Vadala G, Del Vescovo R, et al. T1rho magnetic resonance imaging quantification of early lumbar intervertebral disc degeneration in healthy young adults. Spine (Phila Pa 1976) 2012; 37:1224–30.

# Works Cited

1. **Jung, Carl G.** *Modern Man in Search of a Soul.* s.l. : Harcourt Harvest, 1955 5th Edition p. 234.

2. *Relieving Pain in America: A Blueprint for Transforming Prevention, Care, Education, and Research.* s.l. : IOM, 2001 p.1.

3. **Sarno, John E.** *Healing Back Pain.* New York : Warner Brothers, 1991 p. x.

4. —. The Divided Mind: The Epidemic of Mindbody Disorders [6:12]. s.l. : CDM Studios, June 2009.

5. —. [Online] http://www.medscape.com/viewarticle/478840.

6. —. *Healing Back Pain.* New York : Warner Brothers, 1991 p.81.

7. **Jung, Carl G.** *Civilization in Transition.* s.l. : Princeton University Press, 1970 2nd Edition; Volume 10:153.

8. **Sarno, John E.** *The Mindbody Prescription.* New York : Warner Brothers, 1999 p.141.

9. *Visually Assessed Severity of Lumbar Spinal Canal Stenosis Is Paradoxically Associated With Leg Pain and Objective Walking Ability.* **Pekka Kuittinen, Petri Sipola, Tapani Saari, Timo Juhani Aalto, Sanna Sinikallio, Sakari Savolainen, Heikki Kroger, Veli Turunen, Ville Leinonen, Olavi Airaksinen.** 15:348, s.l. : BMC Musculosketal Disorders, 2014.

10. *Magnetic Resonance Imaging of the Lumbar Spine in People Without Back Pain.* **Maureen C Jensen, Michael N Brant-Zawadzki, Nancy Obuchowski, Michael T Modig, Dennis Malkasian, and Jeffrey S Ross.** 2, s.l. : New England Journal of Medicine, 1994, Vol. 331.

11. *Systematic Literature Reveiw of Imaging Features of Spinal Degeneration in Asymptomatic Populations.* **W Brinjikji, PH Luetmer, B Comstock, BW Bresnahan, LE Chen, RA Deyo, S Halabi, JA Turner, AL Avins, K James, JT Wald, KF Kallmes, and JG Jarvik.** s.l. : American Journal of Neurology, Vol. doi:10.3174/ajnr.A4173.

12. *All the Rage.* Rumur Films, 2014: Film In Production.

13. **Sarno, John E.** *The Mindbody Prescription.* New York : Warner Brothers, second cover, 1999.

14. **Siedle, Edward.** America's Best Doctor and His Miracle Cures: Dr. John E. Sarno. *Forbes Magazine.* 2012, September 26.

15. **Jung, Carl G.** *Analytical Psychology: Its Theory & Practice.* s.l. : Vintage, 1970.

16. *The global burden of musculoskeletal conditions for 2010: an overview of methods.* **DG Hoy, E Smith, M Cross, L Sanchez-Riera, R Buchbinder, FM Blyth, P Brooks, AD Woolf, RH Osborne, M Fransen, T Driscoll, JD Blore, C Murray, N Johns, M Naghavi, E Carnahan, LM March.** 6:982-9, s.l. : Annals of Rheumatic Diseases, 2014, Vol. 73.

17. **Welch, H. Gilbert.** Why the Best Doctors Often Do Nothing. *The Wall Street Journal.* 2015, March 25.

18. **Dubos, Rene.** *Man Adapting.* s.l. : Yale University Press, 1966. ISBN 0-300-00437-0.

19. [Video] s.l. : Good News Broadcast, 2010. http://www.youtube.com/watch?v=9ymsLSiA2RA.

20. **Sarno, John E.** *The Mindbody Prescription: Healing the Body, Healing the Pain.* s.l. : Warner Books, 1998. p. Back Cover. ISBN 0-446-52076-4.

21. **Hanscom, David.** https://www.youtube.com/watch?v=9g2TUqwSoBA. [Online]

22. **Rajaee SS, Bae HW, Kanim LE, Delamarter RB.** *PubMed.* [Online] Jan 1, 2012. [Cited: Jun 6, 2016.] http://www.ncbi.nlm.nih.gov/pubmed/21311399.

23. **Brook I Martin, Anna NA Tosteson, Jon D Lurie, Sohail K Mirza, Philip R Goodney, Nino Dzebiasashvili, David C Goodman, Kristen K Bronner.** *Variaion in the Care of Surgical Conditions: Spinal Stenosis.* s.l. : The Dartmouth Institute, 2014.

24. Back in Control. [Online] November 24, 2013. [http://www.drdavidhanscom.com/2013/11/am-i-operating-on-your-pain-or-anxiety/].

25. **Hutschnecker, Arnold.** *The Will to Live; Your mind - Your health - and You.* New York : Permabooks, 1956. pp. 71-72.

26. *Why Most Published Research Findings Are False.* **Ioannidis, John P. A.** s.l. : PLoS Med 2(8): e124, 2005 Aug.

27. **Alex T Baria, Marwan N Baliki, Thomas J Schnitzer, and Apkar Vania Apkarian.** Wiley Online Library. [Online] October 12, 2014. http://onlinelibrary.wiley.com/doi/10.1002/hbm.22656/abstract.

28. **Weil, Andrew.** *Spontaneous Healing.* s.l. : Random House, 1995.

29. **Harkin, Tom.** Chronic Pain Treatment. s.l. : C-SPAN2, February 14, 2012.

30. **Jung, Carl G.** Concerning Rebirth. *The Collected Works of CG Jung.* Princeton : Princeton University Press, 1939.

31. *New York Times.* [Online] 2008. http://www.nytimes.com/2008/11/11/health/11real.html?_r=1.

32. [Online] http://www.earthrangers.com/wildwire/risk/polar-bears-have-clear-hair-so-why-so-they-look-white/.

33. *Effects of Step-wise Increases in Dietary Carbohydrate on Circulating Saturated Fatty Acids and Palmitoleic Acid in Adults with Metabolic Syndrome.* **Brittanie M Volk, Laura J Kunces, Daniel J Freidenreich, Brian R Kupchak, Catherine Saenz, Juan C Artistizabal, Maria Luz Fernandez, Richard S Bruno, Carl M Maresh, William J Kraemer, Stephen D Phinney, Jeff S Volek.** s.l. : PLOS ONE, 2014, Vol. DOI: 10.1371/journal.pone.011360.

34. *Acupuncture for Chronic Knee Pain, A Randomized Clinical Trial.* **Rana S Hinman, Paul McCrory, Marie Pirotta, Ian Relf, Andrew Forbes, Kay M Crossley, Elizabeth Williamson, Mary Kyriakides, Kitty Novy, Ben R Metcalf, Anthony Harris, Prasuna Reddy, Philip G Conaghan, and Kim L Bennell.** 13, s.l. : Journal of the American Medical Society, 2014, Vol. 312.

35. **Bullpooky, Hippy Dippy.** *Amazon.com book review.* May 12, 2015.

36. *Psychological Variables in Human Cancer.* **Klopfer, Bruno.** 1957, Journal of Projective Techniques, Vol. 21, pp. 331-340.

37. **Helen Schucman, William Thetford.** s.l. : The Foundation for Parasensory Investigation , 1975.

38. **Bray, Libba.** *The Sweet Far Thing.* s.l. : Ember, 2009. ISBN-10: 0440237777.

39. *Comparison of Internal Mammary Artery Ligation and Sham Operation for Angina Pectoris.* **EG Diamond, CF Kittle, JE Crockett.** 4: 483-486, s.l. : American Journal of Cardiology, 1960, Vol. 5.

40. **Kallmes, David F.** [Online] http://www.dailymail.co.uk/health/article-2558438/The-remarkable-power-PLACEBO-effect-Patients-FAKE-surtery-broken-recovered-just-documentary-reveals.html.

41. *Arthroscopic Partial Meniscectomy versus Sham Surgery for a Degenerative Meniscal Tear.* **Raine Sihvonen, Mika Paavola, Antti Malmivaara, Ari Itälä, Antti Joukainen, Heikki Nurmi, Juha Kalske, and Teppo L.N. Järvinen.** s.l. : New England Journal of Medicine, 2013, Vols. 369:2515-2524.

42. **Cabot, Richard.** Truth and Falsehood in Medicine. s.l. : The St. Louis Medical Review, 1903. Vol. 47:208.

43. **Harvey, Shannon.** *The Connection.* [prod.] Harriet Archibald. Elemental Media , 2014.

44. **Siegel, Bernie S.** *Love, Medicine, and Miracles: Lessons Learned about Self-Healing from a Surgeon's Experience with Exceptional Patients.* s.l. : Quill, 1986.

45. *Laughter is the Best Medicine: And it's a great adjunct in the treatment of patients with cancer.* **Patillo, Charlene G. S., Itano, Joanne.** April 2001, American Journal of Nursing, Vol. 101, pp. 40-43.

46. **Thompson, Dawn.** Dancer who suffered years of agonising back pain cured using the lid from a honey jar. *Dailyrecord.co.uk.* [Online] Daily Record and Sunday Mail, May 2, 2016.

47. **Goleman, Daniel.** New Focus on Multiple Personality. *The New York Times - Science.* [Online] May 21, 1985.

48. **Hutschnecker, Arnold.** *The Will to Live.* New York : Thomas Y Crowell Co, 1951.

49. **Jung, Carl G.** Psychology and Religion:West and East. *Collected Works 11: Psychology and Religion.* s.l. : Yale University, 1938.

50. **Cromie, William J.** Computer use deleted as carpal tunnel syndrome cause. *Harvard Gazette.* February 2, 2006.

51. *Multidisciplinary Biopsychosocial Rehabilitation for Chronic Low Back Pain.* **SJ Kamper, AT Apeldoorn, A Chiarotto, RJ Smeets, RW Ostelo, J Guzman, MW van Tulder.** s.l. : The Cochrane Database of Systemic Reviews, 2014, Vol. doi: 10.1002/14651858.

52. [Online] http://www.cochrane.org/CD000963/BACK_multidisciplinary-treatment-for-back-pain.

53. **Eddy, Mary Baker.** *Science and Health With Key to the Scriptures.* s.l. : First Church of Christ, Boston, 1994. 1147252009.

54. [Online] http://www.nytimes.com/2008/01/14/health/14pain.html?pagewanted=all&_r=0.

55. **Berenson, Alex.** Drug Approved. Is Disease Real? *The New York Times.* 2008, January 14.

56. **Beardsley, Allison.** TMS Healing Wall of Victory - Testimonial Block # 13 - Allison. s.l. *www.youtube.com.* [Online] [Cited: June 9, 2016.]

57. **Rath, Marc.** Bristol woman "killed herself after benefits were stopped". *Bristol Post.* 2013, November 25.

58. **Einstein, Albert.** 'The Real Problem Is in the Hearts of Men'; Professor Einstein says a new type of thinking is needed to meet the challenge of the atomic bomb. s.l. : New York Times Magazine, June 23, 1946.

59. **Quint, Michael.** Bane of Insurers: New Ailments. *New York Times.* November 28, 1994.

60. **Evanoff, Bradley A.** Whatever Happened to the Carpal Tunnel Epidemic? [interv.] Suzie Lechtenberg. *Freakonomics Radio.* September 12, 2013.

61. *Why Carpal Tunnel Cases are Plummeting.* [Online] New York : NBCNews.com, 2008.

62. **Craig, Dr. Edward V.** *What ever happened to carpal tunnel? .* [Online] s.l. : NBCNews.com, 2008.

63. **Monica L Wolford, Kathleen Palso, and Anita Bercovitz.** Hospitalization for Total Hip Replacement Among Inpatients Ated 45 and Over: United States, 2000-2010. *National Center for Health Statistices.* 2015, 186.

64. **Sopher, Marc D.** *To Be or Not to Be ... Pain-Free: The Mindbody Syndrom.* Boston : 1st Books Library, Edition 1, pages 106-107, 2003.

65. **Sarno, John E.** Healing Back Pain. s.l. : Mumbleypeg Productions, 2000. Vol. Video Lecture.

66. *No stress--no whiplash? Prevalence of "whiplash" symptoms following exposure to a placebo rear-end collision.* **WH Castro, SJ Meyer, ME Becke,CG Nentwig, MF Hein, BI Ercan, SThomann, U Wessels,AE Du Chesne.** s.l. : International Journal of Legal Medicine, 2001, Vols. 114:316-22.

67. **Rankin, Lissa.** *The Shocking Truth About Your Health.* [Video] s.l. : TEDxFiDiWomen, 2014.

68. **Mafi, John.** Why Tracking Health Too Closely Could Actually Work Against You by Carolyn Gregoire. s.l. : Huffington Post, April 15, 2015.

69. **Groddeck, Georg.** *The Book of the It.* New York : Vintage Books, 1949.

70. **Sarno, John E.** *The Divided Mind: The Epidemic of Mindbody Disorders.* s.l. : Harper Perennial, 2007. 0061174300.

71. **Hall, Calvin S.** *A Primer of Freudian Psychology* . s.l. : Plume, 1999. 0452011833.

72. *The Town That Caught Tourette's.* s.l. : The Learning Channel, 2013.

73. **Cousins, Norman.** *Anatomy of an Illness.* s.l. : Bantom, 1981. p. 39.

74. **Sarno, John E.** *Health Talk.* WOR 710, New Yord : Dr. Ronald Hoffman, April 10th, 2007.

75. —. Dr. Sarno's Cure. [interv.] John Stossel. *20/20 with John Stossel.* s.l. : ABC, July 1999.

76. **Kezman, Ales.** TMS Healing Wall of Victory - Testimonial Block #2 - Ales. s.l. : You Tube, January 4, 2016.

77. **Jung, Carl G.** Marriage as a Psychological Relationship. *The Collected Works of C.G. Jung.* Volume 17 : Princeton University Press , 1925.

78. —. Psychology and Alchemy . *The Collected Works of C.G. Jung.* Volume 12 pages 99-100 : Princeton University Press, 1952.

79. —. The Philosophical Tree. [book auth.] Carl G Jung. *The Collected Works of C.G. Jung.* Volume 13 pages 265-266 : Princeton University Press, 1945.

80. *Regulating Compounding Pharmacies after NECC.* **Outterson, Kevin.** s.l. : New England Journal of Medicine, 2012, Vols. 367:1969-1972.

81. **Horney, Karen.** *Self-Analysis.* s.l. : W W Norton & Company, 1942.

82. **Ware, Bronnie.** *The Top Five Regrets of the Dying: A Life Transformed by the Dearly Departing.* s.l. : Hay House, 2012. 9781401940652.

83. *Intrinsic Shape of the Lumbar Spine and its Effect on Lifting Manoeruvres.* **AV Pavlova, JR Meakin, K Cooper, RJ Barr,and RM Aspden.** Supp 4-17, s.l. : Bone Joint Journal, Vol. 96B.

84. Mark Twain's Autograph. *Atlanta Constitution.* September 9, p. E3, 1096.

85. *United States trends in lumbar fusion surgery for degenerative conditions.* **RA Deyo, ET Gray, W Kreuter, S Mirza, BI Martin.** 2005, Spine, Vol. 30, pp. 1441-5.

86. **Sarno, John E.** *The Divided Mind: The Epidemic of Mindbody Disorders.* s.l. : Harper Perennial, 2007. 0061174300.

# Index

Printed in Great Britain
by Amazon

25435781R00128